Case Presentations in Pa

Other titles published

Case Presentations in Renal Medicine

Titles in preparation

Case Presentations in Cardiology
Case Presentations in Chemical Pathology
Case Presentations in Endocrinology
Case Presentations in Gastroenterology

Case Presentations in Paediatrics

Vanda Joss, MRCP
Consultant Paediatrician, Milton Keynes Hospital

Stephen J. Rose, MRCP
Lecturer in Child Health, University of Aberdeen

Butterworths
London Boston Durban Singapore Sydney Toronto Wellington

All rights reserved. No part of this publication may be reproduced or transmitted in any form or by any means, including photocopying and recording, without the written permission of the copyright holder, application for which should be addressed to the Publishers. Such written permission must also be obtained before any part of this publication is stored in a retrieval system of any nature.

This book is sold subject to the Standard Conditions of Sale of Net Books and may not be re-sold in the UK below the net price given by the Publisher in their current price list.

First published, 1983

© Butterworths & Co. (Publishers) Ltd 1983

British Library Cataloguing in Publication Data

Joss, Vanda
   Case presentation in paediatrics.
   1. Pediatrics
   I. Title   II. Rose, Stephen J.
   616.92   RJ45

ISBN 0-407-00234-0

Library of Congress Cataloguing in Publication Data

Joss, Vanda.
   Case presentations in paediatrics.
   Bibliography: p.
   Includes index.
   1. Pediatrics—Case studies.   I. Rose, Stephen J.
   II. Title.
   RJ58.J67   1983   618.92′009   83–18927

ISBN 0-407-00234-0

Photoset by Illustrated Arts, Sutton, Surrey
Printed and bound by Cox and Wyman Ltd (Reading)

Preface

Membership of the appropriate professional college or association of physicians is the last competitive examination for those attempting to scale the slopes of a career in hospital medicine. In the UK, Membership of the Royal College of Physicians (MRCP) Part II is now taken some time into the junior doctor's training, making a change of career difficult should the candidate fail to pass after several attempts. With this in mind we have written this book in the hope that it will help candidates over this particular hurdle.

The 'grey' cases in the written paper carry a significant proportion of marks, and for many they are the most difficult part. Each 'grey' case contains discrete pieces of relevant information, which can be in any part of the question and may be hidden among irrelevant information. It can, therefore, be difficult to sort the wheat from the tares. Our cases have been written in broadly the same format, with (we hope) the same degree of cunning in spreading the relevant facts throughout the question. Some questions are more difficult than those in the examination, some easier; but the mixture will allow the reader to decipher the code of the questions. The topics of the questions do not reflect the frequency of disease; indeed, some cases are extremely rare, but sufficient information is contained in all questions to allow a logical conclusion while precluding an inspired guess.

The book is aimed mainly at those candidates taking paediatric membership, but will also be of benefit to candidates of the adult membership because one of the four cases is usually paediatric. The Diploma of Child Health does not entirely follow the same format as Membership, but the approach of this book should also be useful to these candidates. We hope our book will also be helpful to those studying for equivalent examinations outside the UK.

We would like to thank our colleagues and mentors at Westminster Children's Hospital for their encouragement and constructive criticism, Miss M Correa, Miss R Western and Miss Tracy Malcolm for patiently typing and retyping the manuscript and also our publishers for their patience, tactful cajoling and encouragement during the times we almost despaired.

Vanda Joss
Stephen Rose

1 Case Presentations and Questions

Case 1

A 6-year-old West Indian girl developed swelling of the left knee. She had been well that morning at nursery school, but then complained of pain in her left knee, which subsequently became swollen. There was no history of trauma whilst at nursery school that morning. There had been no recent illnesses, her appetite was good and she did not suffer from diarrhoea. She had had no previous hospital admissions.

Birth was by lower-segment caesarean section (LSCS) as the mother had had two previous LSCS. The neonatal period was normal.

She sat at 7 months, began talking at 11 months and walked at 16 months. She was third-generation British and both parents were West Indian; her father, aged 37 years, was a bus driver and her mother, aged 34 years was an office cleaner. The two older siblings were healthy. The family lived in a three-bedroomed, semi-detached council house.

Examination

Height, 118.3 cm (90th centile).
Weight, 20.1 kg (50th centile).
Not clinically anaemic.
Pyrexial, 37.9 °C orally.
Pulse, 92/min; Blood pressure, 95/60 mm Hg.
Short soft midsystolic ejection murmur.
Breath sounds normal.
Abdomen not tender.
No hepatosplenomegaly.
Bowel sounds normal.
Tonsils enlarged — not infected.
No rash.
Left knee — swollen, inflamed, tender, with restricted movement.

Investigations

Haemoglobin (Hb), 9.2 g. 100 ml^{-1}.
White blood count (WBC), 10.1 × 10^9. ℓ^{-1}.
Neutrophils, 73%; Lymphocytes, 24%; Macrocytes, 2%; Eosinophils, 1%; Platelets, 215 × 10^9. ℓ^{-1}.
X-Ray left knee, soft-tissue swelling.

Questions

1. Give three possible diagnoses.
2. Give two further investigations.

Case 2

A 16-year-old boy is brought to you because of small stature. His parents are fairly sure that growth was much the same as his peers until 8 years of age. His general health has been good, appetite normal and, apart from morning headaches over the past few months, there have been no symptoms and no past history of note. He attends the local secondary school where he is of average ability, but he is not keen on sports.

The father is 178 cm tall and was pubertal about the age of 13 years. The mother is 152.4 cm tall; menarche was at 15 years. There is one 14-year-old male sibling, who is taller than his brother.

Examination

Height, 149 cm (< 3rd centile).
Weight, 34.3 kg (< 3rd centile).
No secondary sexual characteristics, infantile penis, both testes of prepubertal size.
All other systems normal.

Questions

1. What four important investigations would you do?

Case 3

A 3-week-old baby boy was admitted from casualty with vomiting. He had been well until 2 days before admission when he had begun to vomit 4–5 times daily. The vomiting was not related to feeding and was not projectile. The vomitus contained neither blood nor bile and there was no accompanying diarrhoea. The child was breast fed exclusively and any extra fluid given as boiled water.

The pregnancy was normal and terminated spontaneously; forceps were required for the final 'lift out'. Birth weight was 3.462 kg. There were no neonatal problems, breast feeding was established rapidly and he was discharged on day 8. Mother and baby were seen twice weekly by the community midwife, who had reported no problems.

The father was a 24-year-old silversmith; the mother, aged 27 years, had been a nurse before becoming pregnant. This was their first child. They lived in one room in a 'commune' with amenities shared with nine other people.

Examination

Weight, 3.53 kg.
Rectal temperature, 37.8 °C.
Clinically dehydrated with a dry mouth, sunken fontanelle and poor tissue turgor.
Pulse, 164/min; blood pressure, 80/55 mm Hg by Doppler.
Heart sounds, normal.
Respiratory rate, 42/min.
Normal chest sounds.
Abdomen not distended.
Hepar, 1 cm — no splenomegaly.
Bowel sounds, normal.
Rectal examination — normal stool.
Normal male genitalia with both testes descended.
Pupils reacted to light.
Fundi normal.
Tone hypotonic.
Reflexes — normal.
Plantars — extensor.

4

Investigations

A test meal was attempted, but the baby refused the feed; an emergency barium meal, performed whilst haematological investigations were awaited, revealed no pyloric tumour.
Hb, 12.9 g. 100 ml^{-1}.
WBC, $4.3 \times 10^9. \ell^{-1}$.
Sodium, 125 mmol. ℓ^{-1}.
Potassium, 7.1 mmol. ℓ^{-1}.
Bicarbonate, 18 mmol. ℓ^{-1}.
Urea, 12.3 mmol. ℓ^{-1}.
Urinary: 17 hydroxysteroids, 0.8 μmol/24h (normal, 4–24 μmol/24h); 17 oxosteroids, 0.2 μmol/24h (normal, < 7 μmol/24h); Pregnaetriol — nil detected.

Questions

1. What is the most likely diagnosis?

Case 4

An active and otherwise asymptomatic 8-year-old boy has a history of gradual onset of mild pain in the right hip preceded by a mild, febrile illness with coryza. The pain subsided in a few days but recurred 3 months later with aching in the right knee and groin associated with a runny nose and a low-grade fever. His paternal grandparents suffered from osteoarthritis and an aunt from mild rheumatoid arthritis. His siblings, a sister aged 6 and brother aged 11 years, were both well with no similar problems. His mother was pregnant and had just had a threatened miscarriage. His father was a French teacher and in good health.

Examination

Height, 117 cm (10th centile).
Weight, 19.3 cm (10th centile).
Pulse, 96/min; sinus arrythmia.

Blood pressure, 100/60 mm Hg.
Heart sounds, normal — no added sounds.
Right hip: 10 degrees internal rotation, 10 degrees external rotation and 30 degrees abduction.
All other joints, full painless movements.
Gait — limp on right leg.

Investigations

Hb, 11.8 g. 100 ml^{-1}.
Haematocrit, 36%.
WBC, 7.8 × 10^9. ℓ^{-1}; polymorphs, 85%; lymphocytes, 15%.
ESR, 20 mm, in first hour.
Hb electrophoresis, AA.
Latex fixation, negative.
X-ray hips: sclerosis and partial collapse of the right femoral head with loss of the lateral superior quadrant, some cystic changes and slight lateral extrusion of the femoral head from the acetabulum.
Technetium-99 scan, focal decreased activity with surrounding zone of reaction and increased uptake in the right hip.
Bone age, 7 years.

Questions

1. The MOST likely diagnosis is?
2. What two other conditions should be considered in the differential diagnosis?
3. What is the prognosis?

Case 5

A 10-year-old girl presented in the Accident and Emergency Department complaining of constant abdominal pain of 3 days' duration; there were no precipitating or exacerbating factors. Over the past few months she had been drinking up to 5ℓ of fluid daily and waking several times during the night to drink. She was not enuretic and had no dysuria, vulval soreness, headaches or episodes of weakness. There had been no previous episodes or serious illnesses, but she had suffered a head injury recently which had not necessitated hospital admission.

Her adoptive father had recently left work with terminal Hodgkin's disease to be cared for at home. There were two older adopted siblings in the family. Academic progress at school was good although recently her teachers had reported a lack of concentration in class.

Examination

Examination revealed an apyrexial, well-nourished child, not clinically dehydrated, but complaining of thirst.
Height, 131 cm (25th centile).
Weight, 26.4 kg (25th centile).
Pulse, 80/min; sinus arrhythmia; blood pressure, 110/60 mm Hg.
Respirations, 24/min.
Tenderness in the umbilical area, right subcostal area and in both renal angles. No masses palpable.
Visual fields, normal to gross testing. Pupils equal and reacting to light. Fundi normal.
No secondary sexual characteristics.

Investigations

Hb, 12.1 g. 100 ml^{-1}.
WBC, 5.4×10^9. ℓ^{-1}.
Sodium, 134 mmol. ℓ^{-1}.
Potassium, 4.4 mmol. ℓ^{-1}.
Calcium, 2.1 mmol. ℓ^{-1}.
Urinalysis, negative.
After overnight fluid deprivation, the urine osmolality was 496 mosmol. ℓ^{-1}, plasma osmolality 293 mosmol. ℓ^{-1}.

Questions

1. Give three further relevant investigations.
2. What is the most likely diagnosis?

Case 6

A comatose 3-year-old boy is brought to the Accident and Emergency Department by his parents. 2 days previously he had had symptoms of an upper respiratory tract infection with a cough and nasal discharge, which had not been treated with antibiotics. There was no history of croup. On the day of presentation he had vomited several times without diarrhoea and then become comatose. There had not been a marked deterioration in his condition until the episode of vomiting, and he had had no choking episodes associated with the vomiting. There was no blood in the vomitus.

The pregnancy and delivery had been normal and there were no neonatal problems. He was the third child in a family of three; the older siblings were healthy. He had been fully immunized with the exception of pertussis at his parents' request. The father was an international airline pilot; his mother had been an air-hostess until the birth of her first child. The child had not been abroad.

Examination

On examination the child was pyrexial, was not anaemic nor clinically dehydrated.
Pulse, 140/min; blood pressure 90/60 mm Hg. No added heart sounds.
Respiration, 35/min; no added breath sounds.
Comatose — responding to deep pain only; fundi, normal.
Hyper-reflexic; plantars equivocal.
Weight, 13.17 kg (25th centile).
Length, 92.4 cm (25th centile).

Investigations

Hb, 12.3 g. 100 ml^{-1}.
Sodium, 132 mmol. ℓ^{-1}.
Potassium, 3.6 mmol. ℓ^{-1}.
Urea, 5.8 mmol. ℓ^{-1}.
Glucose, 2.9 mmol. ℓ^{-1}.
Lumbar puncture: red blood cells (RBC), 24%; WBC 2×10^6. ℓ^{-1}; lymphocytes; protein, 0.3 g. ℓ^{-1}; glucose, 2.6 mmol. ℓ^{-1}.
Urinalysis, negative.

8

Questions

1. What is the most likely diagnosis?
2. Give two further investigations to elucidate your diagnosis.

Case 7

A 3-year-old child presented in coma. He was born at term following a normal pregnancy. His initial development revealed that he had good head control at 10 weeks. By then he was able to smile. He sat with support at 8 months, and unsupported at 10 months, and walked at 16 months. He babbled and cooed at 8 months and he was able to reach out and grasp toys. He was able to say six words correctly at 18 months. He was not taken to child welfare clinic and was not given vitamins at any time. He was artificially fed throughout and solids were introduced at 2 months. He had regurgitation of food but this was not serious. He was not seen by a doctor for this symptom.

His parents were poor and they lived with the child in an old house with an outside toilet. He was never immunized and the history revealed that he put everything into his mouth. His bowels were normal and his appetite recently had diminished. Over the previous 6 months, behavioural changes had been noticed.

On admission it was learnt that he had convulsed for approximately 45 minutes before stopping spontaneously.

Examination

Height, 84 cm (3rd centile).
Weight, 10.7 kg (3rd centile).
Pyrexial, 38 °C (axilla).
Pale, not clinically anaemic.
Pulse, 112/min; blood pressure, 110/85 mm Hg.
Heart sounds normal — no added sounds.
Responded to painful stimuli and simple commands.
Nuchal rigidity — positive Kernig's sign.
Pupils equal, reacted to light.
Fundoscopy, early bilateral papilloedema; no haemorrhages or exudates.

Diminished tone, upper and lower limbs.
Reflexes, sluggish.
Plantars, flexor.

Questions

1. What is the most likely diagnosis?
2. Give two differential diagnoses.
3. Give three investigations that you would do as soon as possible.

Case 8

A 3-month-old boy is admitted with a 24-hour history of lethargy and 12-hour history of crying, as if in pain, and vomiting. He had been a full-term normal delivery, birth weight 3.2 kg, breast fed with no previous history of note. There was one healthy 17-month-old male sibling and no significant family history.

On examination, his temperature was 39.3 °C and weight on the 90th centile; he was miserable but with no focal signs.

Investigations

Hb, 12.9 g. 100 ml^{-1}.
WBC, 14.9 × 10^9. ℓ^{-1}; polymorphs, 51%; lymphocytes, 47%.
Sodium, 131 mmol. ℓ^{-1}.
Potassium, 4.6 mmol. ℓ^{-1}.
Urea, 4.3 mmol. ℓ^{-1}.
Glucose, 7.2 mmol. ℓ^{-1}.
Cerebrospinal fluid (CSF) — blood-stained sample: microscopy, RBC, 1000 × 10^6. ℓ^{-1}; WBC, 5 × 10^6. ℓ^{-1} lymphocytes (lymphs), 0 neutrophils.
Culture no growth.
Glucose, 5.5 mmol. ℓ^{-1}.
Protein, 1.4 g. ℓ^{-1}; albumin, 2.3 g. ℓ^{-1}; IgG, 0.17 g. ℓ^{-1}.
Bag urine: micros; WBC, 1000 mm^3; culture, *E.coli* > 100 000 organisms/ml, ampicillin resistant, co-trimoxazole sensitive.
Blood culture, no growth.

He was started on ampicillin prior to the sensitivity results, but 2 days later changed to co-trimoxazole. A repeat urine culture the same day yielded: micros; WBC, 20 mm^3; culture < 10 000 organisms/ml.

The temperature initially appeared to be settling, but after 2 days on co-trimoxazole it rose again to 39.5 °C and he was very irritable with vomiting. Again nothing could be found on examination apart from mild meningism.

Repeat septic screen: Throat swab, scanty *E.coli*; nose swab, no growth; stool, no pathogens grown; blood culture, no growth.
Urine: micros; WBC, 5 mm^3; scanty RBC; scanty epithelial cells; culture; < 10 000 organisms/ml.
CSF: slightly turbid cells; 27×10^6 lymphs. ℓ^{-1}, 360×10^6 neuts. ℓ^{-1}, 10×10^6 RBC. ℓ^{-1}; smear, no organisms seen; culture, no growth; protein, 0.78. ℓ^{-1}; sugar, 3.3 mmol. ℓ^{-1}.
Blood sugar, 5.1 mmol. ℓ^{-1}.
Urea electrolytes, normal.
Hb, 10.1 g.100 ml^{-1}.
WBC, 18.3×10^9. ℓ^{-1}; polymorphs 62%; lymph 26%; monocytes 10%.
Film, toxic granulation.
Chest X-ray, normal.

He was treated for meningitis with penicillin and chloramphenicol, but the temperature continued to swing and 2 days later a large mass was felt on the right side of the abdomen. Repeat lumbar puncture confirmed improvement in the CSF cell count.

Questions

1. What two investigations would you do at this stage to aid diagnosis?
2. What is the most likely diagnosis?
3. What two lines of action would you take?

Case 9

A 10-year-old spina bifida boy was admitted from Outpatients with a pathological fracture of his left femur.

He had had an open lumber myelomeningocoele closed on day 1. A muscle chart at this time demonstrated absent lower-limb muscle tone, tendon reflexes and anal reflex absent. Sequential head circumference measurements demonstrated rapid enlargement and a ventriculoperitoneal shunt was inserted at 4 months of age. The distal catheter was lengthened at 18 months and 5 years. At 8 years the proximal catheter was replaced with difficulty and he began to convulse postoperatively.

He was controlled immediately by a mannitol infusion, but began fitting again 3 days postoperatively, requiring long-term phenobarbitone therapy. He had been well since discharge.

Social History:

His parents had been unable to cope with the demands of a handicapped child and had placed him at a Dr Barnardo's home at 2½ years. He had not seen them since.

He attended the remedial class of the local junior school and was considered of below average intelligence.

Examination

Weight, 32.1 kg (90th centile).
Height, 134.4 cm (50th centile).
Pulse, 84/min; blood pressure, 115/75 mm Hg.
Heart sounds, normal.
Peripheral pulses, present.
Chest, thoracic scoliosis.
Breath sounds, normal.
No hepatosplenomegaly.
Palpable faeces, sigmoid colon.
Bladder, palpable.
Rectal examination, faeces to anal margin.
Occipitofrontal circumference (OFC), 55.2 cm.
Shunt, filled and emptied rapidly.
Tone, power, co-ordination: normal in upper limbs, absent in lower limbs.
Pupils, equal; fundi, normal.
Reflexes: normal in upper limbs, absent in lower limbs; no anal reflex.
Deformity and swelling of left thigh.

Investigations

Hb, 10.7 g. 100 ml.
White cell count, 7.3×10^9. ℓ^{-1}.
Sodium, 131 mmol. ℓ^{-1}.
Potassium, 4.1 mmol. ℓ^{-1}.
Calcium, 2.2 mmol. ℓ^{-1}.
Urea, 3.6 mmol. ℓ^{-1}.
Phosphate, 0.97 mmol. ℓ^{-1}.
Alkaline phosphatase, 875 IU. ℓ^{-1}.
Intravenous pyelogram (IVP):
sequential series demonstrating worsening hydronephrosis and dilated ureters.

Questions

1. What is the most likely cause of the diagnosis?
2. What is the treatment?

Case 10

A 12-year-old girl is admitted to hospital with burns on her legs, which she obtained while playing near a bonfire on November 5th. The burns were treated with dry dressings and started to heal. While in hospital it was noted that her behaviour was 'odd'. Her concentration span was very poor, she would suddenly change her attention from one conversation and shout something to another patient. On one occasion she had been walking a little unsteadily across the ward when she fell for no apparent reason. Another time she had fallen out of bed.

She was the third child in a family of four. All other siblings were alive and well, there was no family history of note. The parents had been divorced 18 months earlier; the patient had been distressed at this and still saw her father regularly. Her behaviour had been unpredictable since the summer and in view of this she had been sent to stay with an aunt and uncle for some weeks during the holiday. At school decreasing concentration had led to a deterioration in performance.

In the past she had had tonsillectomy aged 6 years and the usual childhood illnesses including mumps, measles and more recently chickenpox.

Examination

Chest, cardiovascular system and abdomen — normal.
Neurological examination hampered by patients' lack of concentration.
Cranial nerves, intact.
Fundi, normal.
She would suddenly grimace and have jerky movements of the limbs or the whole body. While trying co-ordination tests, movement was slow, but there was no tremor, only occasional odd posturing of the limbs. Movements of limbs were full and tone difficult to assess, but possibly slightly increased in the legs; there was no cogwheeling. Reflexes were all brisk and equal with an extensor plantar on the right, equivocal on the left. Gait was jerky and somewhat unsteady, with heel – toe walking and Romberg's impossible.

Investigations

Hb, 12.3 mg. 100 ml^{-1}.
WBC, 6.7×10^9. ℓ^{-1}; normal differential.
ESR, 26 mm.
Skull X-ray, normal.

Questions

1. What is the diagnosis?
2. What two further investigations would you do?

Case 11

An 18-month-old Ghanaian girl with known sickle-cell disease was admitted to hospital with a pyrexia. She had had a temperature for 3 days, associated with a cough and occasional vomiting. She had always lived in England and her parents were unrelated. Mother was at teacher's training college and left the child with a baby-minder during the day. Father was studying engineering. The only regular medication the child took was folic acid.

Examination

Pale, miserable child — pyrexial, 38.3 °C (axilla).
No jaundice.
Pulse, 124/min; blood pressure, 85/50 mm Hg.
Soft systolic murmur, left sternal border.
Respiratory rate, 30/min.
Breath sounds, normal.
Fauces, inflammed.
Tonsillar nodes, palpable — small, non-tender.
Tympanic membranes, normal.
Liver, 1 cm below costal margin.
Spleen, tipped.
Central nervous system, normal.

Investigations

Hb, 8.3 g. 100 ml^{-1}.
WBC, 22.7 × 10^9. ℓ^{-1}; polymorphs (polys), 63%; lymphs, 31%; monocytes (monos), 4%; eosinophils (eosin.), 2%.
Urea, 5.4 mmol. ℓ^{-1}.
Sodium, 139 mmol. ℓ^{-1}; potassium, 3.7 mmol. ℓ^{-1}; bicarbonate, 22 mmol. ℓ^{-1}.
Throat-swab culture, normal mouth commensals.
Mid-stream urine (MSU): micros. WBC 13 mm^3; Culture, < 10 000 organisms/ml.
Urinalysis, nothing abnormal detected (NAD).
Blood culture, no growth.
Chest X-ray, some consolidation in the right middle lobe.

She was treated with penicillin intramuscularly because of the vomiting and the temperature settled after 24 hours. Penicillin V was then substituted but she again became pyrexial. It was thought that she was not taking the medication properly from mother and intramuscular penicillin was thus restarted. Again the temperature settled, but on changing back to penicillin V she became pyrexial within 24 hours. She continued to sit on her mother's lap, very miserable, withdrawn and anorexic. No new physical signs could be found on examination.

Questions

1. What three investigations would you do immediately?
2. What is the most likely diagnosis?
3. What is the treatment?

Case 12

A 9-year-old boy is referred to the Gastroenterology Outpatients by his general practitioner for investigation of chronic diarrhoea of 7 weeks' duration. He had been treated with antibiotics and antidiarrhoeal agents to no avail and was now beginning to lose weight.

The diarrhoea started 2 weeks after a Crusader camping holiday in Guernsey and, since then, he had passed loose stools three or four times daily. The diarrhoea was not obviously exacerbated by any foodstuffs and was not accompanied by abdominal pain, tenesmus or pain on defaecation. His appetite was still good. The stools were not frothy, flushed away easily and contained no blood or mucus. He had had no previous similar episodes and no one else in the family was affected.

On systems analysis he admitted to the occasional headache which was mild, frontal, had no aura and resolved rapidly. The only previous medical problem was an admission following a road traffic accident.

His school reports were above average and he had been made class captain for that year. His older brother had been elected school captain. His father was a successful 46-year-old merchant banker; his mother was 35 years old and a part-time freelance journalist. They lived in a large, luxurious detached house in Suburbia.

Examination

Pleasant, intelligent co-operative child.
Height, 133.2 cm (50th centile).
Weight, 24.2 kg (10th centile).
Pulse, 88/min; blood pressure, 140/100 — checked twice.

16

Apex beat not displaced.
Heart sounds, normal.
Peripheral pulses, normal.
Abdomen not distended; no hepatosplenomegaly.
Rectal examination — empty rectum.
Genitalia — normal pre-pubertal.
Pupils reacted to light; fundi, discs normal.
Tone, power and co-ordination normal.
Reflexes normal.

Investigations

Hb, 12.3 g. 100 ml^{-1}.
Mean cell volume (MCV), 80 fl.
Mean cell haemoglobin (MCH), 29 pg.
Mean cell haemoglobin concentration (MCHC), 32 g. dl^{-1}.
WBC, 7.5×10^9. ℓ^{-1}; neuts, 54%; lymphs, 43%; monos, 2%; eosin., 1%.
Sodium, 138 mmol. ℓ^{-1}.
Potassium, 3.2 mmol. ℓ^{-1}.
Calcium, 2.46 mmol. ℓ^{-1}.
Phosphate, 1.35 mmol. ℓ^{-1}.
Bicarbonate, 24 mmol. ℓ^{-1}.
Urea, 2.0 mmol. ℓ^{-1}.
Stools for giardiasis and bacteriology, negative.
Barium enema, normal.
MSU × 3, negative culture.
IVP, normal.
ECG, normal.

Whilst in hospital his blood pressure settled at 125/90 mm Hg and his diarrhoea responded to antidiarrhoeal agents. He was discharged with a month's outpatient appointment.

At this appointment he was noted to have ptosis and meiosis of the left eye with loss of sweating on the ipsilateral side of his face.

Questions

1. What is the most likely diagnosis?
2. Give two further important investigations?

Case 13

An 11-year-old girl who has had nephrotic syndrome since the age of 20 months presents in relapse for the twelfth time. She has always been steriod responsive and had highly selective proteinuria with a normal serum complement. A renal biopsy at the age of 2 years was consistent with minimal change disease. She had a 6-week course of cyclophosphamide when 4 years old and was then relapse free for 4 years. Her last relapse had been 9 months previously and she had been off steriods for 3 months.

She had a history of proteinuria and oedema 5 days prior to this admission, but for the previous 24 hours she had had severe abdominal pain, vomiting and dizziness on standing up.

Examination

Height, 132.7 cm (10th centile).
Weight, 45.2 kg (75th centile).
Apyrexial.
Oedema of ankles and face.
Pulse, 92/min — sinus arrhythmia; blood pressure, 85/60 mm Hg.
Heart sound, normal.
Chest clear.
Abdomen — not distended, diffusely tender, bowel sounds present.

Investigations

Hb, 12.6 g. 100 ml^{-1}.
WBC, 7.6 × 10^9. ℓ^{-1}.
Sodium, 136 mmol. ℓ^{-1}.
Potassium, 4.2 mmol. ℓ^{-1}.
Bicarbonate, 21 mmol. ℓ^{-1}.
Urea, 6.0 mmol. ℓ^{-1}.
Total protein, 54 g. ℓ^{-1}.
Albumin, 14 g. ℓ^{-1}.
24-hour urine, 9.5. (g protein)$^{-1}$.
Blood culture, throat swab — no growth.

Following admission she continued to vomit copiously up to 11 times daily. She continued to drink and pass 300 ml urine per day with heavy proteinuria but still felt faint although her abdominal pain improved. 3 days later she complained of pain in her legs. On examination she had lost 1.2 kg in weight, there was still very minimal oedema, blood pressure 100/80 mm Hg. Her peripheries were cool, especially her feet which were cold with loss of fine touch sensation and movement. The calf and thigh muscles were tender bilaterally. Peripheral pulses wer present but decreased at the wrist, the femorals were weak, but neither popliteals nor dorsalis pedis pulses could be felt. Heart sounds were normal and the chest clear. Her abdomen was a little distended and tender.

Repeat investigations:

Sodium, 133 mmol. ℓ^{-1}.
Potassium, 5.1 mmol. ℓ^{-1}.
Bicarbonate, 16 mmol. ℓ^{-1}.
Urea, 19 mmol. ℓ^{-1}.
Albumin, 5 g./ℓ^-.
Hb, 15 g. 100 ml$^-$.
WBC, 27.0×10^9. ℓ^{-1}.
Platelets, 179×10^9. ℓ^{-1}.

Questions

1. What are the two most important pathologies to consider?
2. What three investigations would you do immediately?
3. What three lines of treatment would you start?

Case 14

An 8-year-old boy diagnosed as a diabetic 10 months previously has been controlled on a daily dose of 16 units Monotard insulin. Initially control was satisfactory, but 3 months ago he developed morning glycosuria at more than 2% associated with ketonuria. During the day there was usually 0–½% glycosuria. Both mother and child were very careful with his injection dose and sites, diet and urine tests. Over the last 3 months, the Monotard insulin dose had been gradually increased to 28 units with no improvement in control. The glycolysated Hb (Hb AIC) was low.

Questions

1. What is the most likely cause for the glycosuria and ketonuria?
2. What would be the most helpful investigation?
3. In what two ways would you alter management?

Case 15

A 32-year-old single Jamaican mother, who has had four previous miscarriages between 12 and 16 weeks' gestation, had a forceps delivery of a 30 week' gestation female infant weighing 1.3 kg. At birth the baby required intubation for 4 min, Apgar scores were 2 at 1 min, 10 at 10 mins. The membranes had been ruptured for 32 hours and mother had had three doses of betamethasone. She had been pyrexial just before delivery and was treated with ampicillin. *Staphylococcus aureus* was grown from her high vaginal swab.

On examination the baby was a normal female infant, consistent with 30 weeks' gestation.

Investigations at birth:

Hb, 15.1 g. 100 ml^{-1}.
WBC, 6.2 × 10^9. ℓ^{-1}.
Gastric aspirate, Gram positive cocci seen.
Blood culture, no growth.
All surface swabs, *Staph. aureus* grown.

The baby was given flucloxacillin and gentamicin for 1 week. Mild jaundice, not requiring phototherapy, was the only problem.

Table 1
Serial blood on automated machine

Age (Days)	Hb (g. 100 ml^{-1})	Total WBC (× 10^9. ℓ^{-1})	Polys (%)	Platelets
1	15.1	7.3		Normal
4	17.0	10.1		Normal
11	13.2	34.1		Normal
18	8.3	50.5	3	Normal

Infection screen, no significant growth.
Mother and baby's blood group, both 'B' +ve.
Immunoglobulins, within normal limits for prematurity.

Questions

1. What two further investigations would you do?
2. What is the most likely explanation of this blood count?

Case 16

A 31-year-old Danish woman was admitted in established labour after falling on ice during a Christmas shopping trip to London. By dates she was 36–37 weeks' gestation; fundal height correlated with this estimation. 18 hours later she was delivered of a healthy female infant weighing 2.624 kg. No resuscitation procedures were necessary. The infant was put to the breast and sucked immediately. The following day she was seen by the paediatric senior house officer, who noted genital abnormalities.

The pregnancy had been uneventful and the mother had taken analgesics only for the occasional headache. No other drugs had been prescribed. This was their second child; the first, a male, had died aged 2 weeks of gastroenteritis.

The father, aged 32 years, owned a campsite just outside Copenhagen; the mother, 31-years, helped with the administration. They lived in a spacious mobile house on the site.

Examination

Weight, 2.590 kg.
Pulse, 142 beats/min.
Heart sounds, normal.
Peripheral pulses, normal.
Respiratory rate, 42 per minute.
Breath sounds, normal.
Liver, 1 cm; no splenomegaly.
Bowel sounds, normal — patent anus.
Genitalia — enlarged clitoris, fused labial folds.

Questions

1. Give two further important examination details.
2. What is the single most important diagnosis? And why?
3. Give two relevant investigations to the above diagnosis.

Case 17

A girl, aged 4 years and 2 months, was rushed to Accident and Emergency by ambulance, unconscious and convulsing. The convulsions were controlled immediately by intravenous diazepam, but the child became apnoeic, requiring mechanical ventilation.

The mother reported that the child had been well that morning, eaten a hearty breakfast and was playing with a friend when she became drowsy and then unconscious. The ambulance was called immediately.

The child had been previously healthy, with no major illnesses or previous hospital admissions. The only drugs in the house were aspirin and Junior Dispirin, kept in a locked bathroom cabinet. The family lived in a modernized thatched cottage, with new plumbing, in a small village. The father, aged 34 years, was headmaster at the local school; the mother, aged 29 years, had not worked since the marriage. Previously she had been a nursing auxilliary. She said she had felt quite depressed since the birth of her second child, now aged 3 months.

Examination

Height, 95.2 cm (10th centile).
Weight, 13.7 kg (40th centile).
Temperature, 36.1 °C.
Pulse, 142/min; blood pressure, 80/50 mm Hg.
Heart sounds, normal.
No spontaneous respiratory movement.
Tympanic membranes, normal.
Throat and larynx normal at intubation.
No abdominal masses.
Pupils dilated, poorly responsive to light.
Deep tendon reflexes, sluggish.
Plantars, downgoing.

Investigations

Hb, 11.9 g. 100 ml^{-1}.
WBC, 5.7 × 10^9. ℓ^{-1}.
Sodium, 131 mmol. ℓ^{-1}.
Potassium, 3.9 mmol. ℓ^{-1}.
Calcium, 2.38 mmol. ℓ^{-1}.
Phosphate, 1.81 mmol. ℓ^{-1}.

Urea, 3.1 mmol. ℓ^{-1}.
Blood cultures × 3, negative.
CSF: 4 lymphs; 244 × 10^6. RBC ℓ^{-1}.
Salicylate level — none detected.
Blood lead, 0.9 μmol. ℓ^{-1}.
Urinalysis, negative.
Amino acid screen, normal.
ECG, atrial tachycardia — no abnormal complexes.
Chest, X-ray clear.

The child was weaned from the ventilator over the next 18 hours and regained full consciousness 36 hours after admission. No neurological sequelae were detected and the patient was discharged 5 days later with no diagnosis. EEG 6 weeks later was normal, but in the follow-up outpatients she was noted to be drowsy, uncoordinated and walking with a wide-based gait. She was re-admitted and over the subsequent 90 minutes developed jerking of her left arm and leg. She recovered over the next 14 hours and was discharged 2 days later; all investigations, including a CT scan, were normal. Over the following 8 weeks she was admitted twice with a similar clinical picture; both times she recovered rapidly with no ill effects. She was then admitted deeply unconscious and fitting. Again mechanical ventilation was required; supraventricular tachycardia developed which rapidly proceeded to ventricular fibrillation; resuscitation was unsuccessful.

Post-mortem revealed no macroscopic abnormalities.

Questions

1. What vital investigation was omitted?

Case 18

A 13-year-old boy is admitted unconscious to hospital having been pulled out of a swimming pool. He had been well and attended school that morning. He had eaten school lunch normally and an hour later gone swimming with the rest of his class. His teacher was uncertain about what had happened. He had been seen diving into the pool and possibly collided with another pupil whilst swimming. He was next seen at the side of the pool, got out, then fell back into it. After being pulled out of the pool he was sat up on the edge by friends, spluttered and momentarily shook all four limbs. An ambulance was called immediately.

He had been born by normal delivery at 42 weeks gestation following induced labour. There were no perinatal problems. He had had mumps, scarlatina, chickenpox then shingles 4 years later. He had recently changed school, but was said to be doing well. His father had died 10 years ago from rheumatic heart disease; his mother was well, supporting the family working as a nurse. She occasionally felt depressed and had difficulty sleeping. There was one brother, aged 11 years, who had broken his arm the day before.

On arrival he was unconscious and responding well to pain but immediately started shaking both arms and legs in a fine tremor. There were no tonic or clonic movements. His head was arched back and he was said to go blue. A pharyngeal airway was inserted but 1 minute later it was coughed up and his colour improved. Following this he became alternately restless and drowsy; he did not respond to commands.

Examination

Apyrexial.
No obvious signs of injury.
Pulse, 72/minute; regular; blood pressure 90/70 mm Hg.
Heart sounds, normal.
Chest — no added sounds.
Abdomen, normal.
No meningism.
Pupils equal — reacted to light; fundoscopy, normal; eye movements, normal.
Cranial nerves, normal as far as tested.
All limbs moved equally.
Tone, increased but equal.
Reflexes, normal.
Plantars, flexor.

Investigations

Hb, 13.7 g. 100 ml^{-1}.
WBC, 10.4 × 10^9. ℓ^{-1}; 52% neuts, 44% lymphs, 4% monos.
Film, normal.
Sodium, 117 mmol. ℓ^{-1}.
Potassium, 5.0 mmol. ℓ^{-1}.
Urea, 3.5 mmol. ℓ^{-1}.
Osmolality, 289 mmol. ℓ^{-1}.
Glucose, 5.4 mmol. ℓ^{-1}.
Skull X-ray, NAD.
Chest X-ray, NAD.

Questions

1. What four diagnoses would you consider first?
2. What four further investigations would you carry out?

Case 19

A 5-month-old baby presents with a rash and pyrexia of 40.5 °C. He had had a mild upper respiratory tract infection and watery eyes 5 days before, followed by a macular erythematous rash on the forehead and trunk with a pyrexia of 37.5 °C. A diagnosis of rubella was made. The rash gradually spread to the limbs and cheeks. He had refused all bottle feeds that day, screamed when a bottle was put in his mouth and on handling, and had had six loose, green motions.

In the past there was no history of note; the parents were unmarried but living together in rented accommodation. He was their first child and appeared well cared for.

Examination

Length, 64.8 cm (25th centile).
Weight, 7.3 kg (50th centile).
Chest cardiovascular system and abdomen — normal.

Pharynx slightly inflammed — mouth clean.
Tympanic membranes, normal.
CNS, normal.
Rash — raised erythematous non-purpuric patches with central white and bluish discoloration on the limbs.
On both calves, few small vesicular lesions.
Face and neck — rash less florid.
Trunk — macular rash.
Marked conjunctivitis with photophobia.
Lips cracked and weeping.

Investigations

Hb, 11.3 g. 100 ml^{-1}.
WBC: 20.9 × 10^9. ℓ^{-1}; 82% polys, 16% lymphs.
Film — toxic granulation of neutrophils.
Urea, 2.2 mmol. ℓ^{-1}.
Sodium, 133 mmol. ℓ^{-1}.
Potassium, 4.0 mmol. ℓ^{-1}.
Blood sugar, 6.0 mmol. ℓ^{-1}.
Throat swab, no growth.
Blood culture, no growth.
Chest X-ray, normal.
CSF: WBC, 21 × 10^6. ℓ^{-1}; lymphs, 18; neutrophils, 3; RBC 0 × 10^6. ℓ^{-1}; Gram's stain, no organism seen; sugar, 3.4 mmol. ℓ^{-1}; protein, 0.26 g. ℓ^{-1}.

Questions

1. What is the diagnosis?
2. What are the four most likely causative agents in this child?
3. What is the usual outcome?

Case 20

A boy, aged 2 years 7 months, is referred from a rural hospital for further treatment of gastroenteritis. He had been admitted 2 days previously, after a 3-day history of vomiting. Oral rehydration had been unsuccessful and, despite intravenous therapy, the child was severely dehydrated on admission. Detailed questioning of the mother revealed that the child had complained of abdominal pain initially and then began forceful vomiting. He had vomited up to five times daily before admission and only slightly less thereafter. The vomitus was bile stained but not bloody. There had been no accompanying diarrhoea and the child had had a normal bowel action the day after admission.

There was a history of two similar episodes 4 and 9 months previously, again with forceful vomiting, but not diarrhoea. The episodes had lasted 3 and 2 days, respectively, and resolved spontaneously.

The pregnancy had been full term and uncomplicated with a home confinement, despite this being the first pregnancy. The child had been breast fed exclusively for 3 months and then weaned. He was fully immunized.

The father was a 26-year-old cowhand; the mother was 22 years old and helped in the farm dairy. They lived in a two-bedroomed tied cottage, with open-fire heating.

Examination

Length, 92.2 cm (25th centile).
Weight, 11.87 kg (10th centile).
No jaundice or anaemia.
The child was apyrexial, had poor tissue turgor and dry mouth.
Pulse, 124/min — poor pulse volume; blood pressure, 80/50 mm Hg.
No added cardiac sounds.
Respiratory rate, 36/min; no added sounds.
Scaphoid abdomen; no hepatosplenomegaly.
Bowel sounds not increased; rectum empty, no blood.
Comatose, responding to handling and pain.
Pupils responded to light; fundi, normal.
Reflexes, sluggish.
Plantars, downgoing.
The child was felt to be approximately 15% dehydrated.

Investigations

Hb, 15.2 g. 100 ml^{-1}.
WBC, 8.7 × 10^9. ℓ^{-1}.

Sodium, 146 mmol. ℓ^{-1}.
Potassium, 3.8 mmol. ℓ^{-1}.
Glucose, 7.3 mmol. ℓ^{-1}.
Urea, 8.9 mmol. ℓ^{-1}.
pH, 7.49.
P_{O_2}, 12.1 kPa.
P_{CO_2}, 5.3 kPa.
Bicarbonate, 32 mmol. ℓ^{-1}.
Base excess, +5 mmol. ℓ^{-1}.
Standard bicarbonate, 29 mmol. ℓ^{-1}.
Standard base excess, +7 mmol. ℓ^{-1}.

Subsequent progress

Half the total of the child's estimated deficit was administered intravenously plus daily requirements as clear fluids over the subsequent 8 hours. The child regained consciousness and began to pass urine. Abdomianl X-ray revealed a dilated stomach and duodenum, with little air distally. No intramural gas was seen.

Questions

1. What is the most likely diagnosis?
2. Give one further useful investigation.

Case 21

A 15-month-old girl is admitted with difficulty in moving her right arm and leg. She had had a mild cold during the previous few days, and on the day before admission the right leg was noticed to collapse under the child on two occasions. On waking up the following morning, she had paralysis of the right side of the body which regressed within a few hours. However, by midday a slight limp of the right leg was noticed. During the course of the afternoon, the parents noticed clonic right-sided seizures associated with mild drowsiness and recurrence of the right-sided paralysis. She had been a full-term, normal delivery, weighing 2.58 kg following a normal pregnancy. She sat at 6 months, walked at 12 months and spoke her first words before 1 year of age. She had had chickenpox and German measles without complications. There were no siblings and no family history of note.

Examination

Height, 77.2 cm (50th centile).
Weight, 10.9 kg (75th centile).
Pyrexial, 37.2 °C (axilla).
Fully conscious.
Subtotal, flaccid right-sided hemiplegia.
Right facial palsy, mainly affecting the lower part of the face.
All other cranial nerves intact.
Decreased right-sided reflexes.
Plantars: right, extensor; left, flexor.

Investigations

Hb, 11.3 g. 100 ml^{-1}.
WBC: 6.8×10^9. ℓ^{-1}; polys, 56%; lymphs, 40%; eosin. 1%; monos, 3%.
Platelets, 246×10^9. ℓ^{-1}.
Prothrombin time, normal.
Blood culture, no growth.
Lumbar puncture — CSF: lymphs, 25×10^6. ℓ^{-1}; polys, 5×10^6. ℓ^{-1}; RBC, 0; protein, 0.1 g. ℓ^{-1}; sugar, 3.4 mmol. ℓ^{-1}.
EEG: polymorphic delta activity over the left hemisphere maximum in the precentral area. Non-specific disturbances over the right hemisphere. Viral studies in stools, CSF and throat washings — negative.

Questions

1. What are the two most likely causes of her hemiplegia?
2. What four investigations would be most helpful at this stage?

Case 22

A 2½-year-old Caucasian girl presents with a 5-week history of increasing pain in the left leg and difficulty walking upstairs. For 2 weeks she has had colicky, abdominal pain with screaming episodes. Over the past 2 days she has developed a temperature and been extremely miserable.

She is an only child, born at term by Keilland's forceps. She was bottle fed and had no neonatal problems apart from mild jaundice. Developmental milestones and growth had been normal. She had been treated twice for otitis media by her general practitioner and had had influenza 2 months previously at the same time as her parents. She does not attend nursery school. Immunizations were given at correct times. Her father is a bus driver; this is his second marriage, he had no children by his previous marriage. Her mother was a secretary in the civil service before the birth of her first child. Finances are a constant problem, even though they live in a two-bedroomed council flat.

On examination she was pyrexial, had some cervical lymphadenopathy, liver 2 cm below the costal margin and the spleen was palpable (2 cm). All of the joints appeared normal.

Investigations

Hb, 9.9 g. 100 ml^{-1}.
WBC, 10.0×10^9. ℓ^{-1}; polys, 1.2×10^9. ℓ^{-1}.
ESR, 58 mm in first hour.
Alkaline phosphatase, 564 IU.
Serum alanine transferase (ALT), 26 IU.
Serum aspartate transferase (AST), 54 IU.

She was treated with aspirin, 100 mg. kg^{-1}. day^{-1} and following this her clinical condition improved, only to deteriorate again a few days later. She was noted to be pale and the repeat blood count was as follows:
Hb, 6 g. 100 ml^{-1}.
WBC, 3.7×10^9. ℓ^{-1}; polys, 2×10^9. ℓ^{-1}.
Platelets, 22×10^9. ℓ^{-1}.
ESR, 93 mm in first hour.

Questions

1. What are three differential diagnoses in order of priority?
2. What six investigations would you do to differentiate?

Case 23

A 17-year-old Spanish girl was admitted to the delivery room in established labour; her membranes had ruptured 14 hours previously. A normal male infant was delivered by breech, requiring no resuscitative procedures.

The mother had lived in England for the past 12 years and had not visited Spain for the past 2 years. She had not attended any antenatal clinics, was unsure of her dates and had smoked approximately 15 cigarettes a day during the pregnancy. The father was a West Indian, who worked as a porter in a meat market. Clinical assessment placed the gestational age of the infant at approximately 33 weeks. Birth weight 1230 g, OFC 27 cm. He was nursed in an incubator and was noted to feed well from a bottle.

At 8 hours of life he suddenly had two apnoeic episodes. Examination after the first episode showed the following: pulse, 140/min. No cyanosis, apyrexial, no jerky movements, fontanelle not bulging and he sucked well.

Investigations

Hb, 16.3 g. 100 ml^{-1}.
WBC, 10.2 × 10^9. ℓ^{-1}; lymphs, 47%; neuts, 50%; monos, 3%.
Platelets, 100 × 10^9. ℓ^{-1}.
Sodium, 138 mmol. ℓ^{-1}.
Potassium, 3.8 mmol. ℓ^{-1}.

Nothing abnormal was detected on further investigation, but despite feeding well and being very active he continued to have short apnoeic episodes.

Questions

1. Give three possible diagnoses.
2. Give four relevant investigations.
3. What is the most likely diagnosis?
4. Give two treatments for the recurrent apnoea.

Case 24

A 5-year-old Asian girl was referred to casualty by her general practitioner with limb weakness. She had been complaining of weakness for 3 days and the general practitioner was then called as she was unable to walk.

4 weeks previously she had contracted chickenpox, but had made an uneventful recovery and had been back at school for 2 weeks. 3 days before presentation she had complained of weakness in her left leg, then the weakness progressed and involved her right leg also. She was now unusually irritable and was complaining of headaches.

She was an active child and participated in sport, but there was no history of injury either during games lessons or in the playground. She was reported to be a co-operative, intelligent child with no behaviour or personality abnormalities.

The medication in the house consisted of Anadin and Andrew's Liver Salts.

The family lived in a two-bedroomed terraced house, with paraffin heating. The father, aged 32 years, was a minicab driver, the mother, aged 26 years, was a seamstress in the local dressmaking factory. There were two healthy siblings, aged 4 and 7 years.

Examination

Height, 99.2 cm, (3rd centile).
Weight, 14.7 kg (3rd centile).

Not clinically anaemic or jaundiced.
Temperature, 38.6 °C.
Pulse, 94/min; sinus arrhythmia.
No added heart sounds.
Enlarged but uninfected tonsils.
No tonsillar nodes.
Abdomen soft, no masses.
No hepatosplenomegaly.
Bowel sounds, normal.
Abdominal reflexes, present.
Neurology — eyes heavily coated in black make-up.
No nuchal rigidity; Kernig's sign negative.
Pupils equal and reacting.
Fundi discs, pink — veins engorged.
Cranials nerve, no abnormalities.
Tone: markedly reduced in left leg; mildly reduced in right leg; arms, normal.
Coordination: both legs, poor; upper limbs, normal.
Sensation: no sensory loss, no joint swelling.
Reflexes: arms, normal; legs, brisk.
Plantars: left, extensor; right, flexor.

Investigations

Hb, 12.7 g. 100 ml^{-1}.
WBC, 13.6 × 10^9. ℓ^{-1}.
Sodium, 133 mmol. ℓ^{-1}.
Potassium, 4.4 mmol. ℓ^{-1}.
Calcium, 2.37 mmol. ℓ^{-1}.
Phosphate, 1.29 mmol. ℓ^{-1}.
Magnesium, 0.77 mmol. ℓ^{-1}.
Glucose, 6.3 mmol. ℓ^{-1}.
Urea, 2.7 mmol. ℓ^{-1}.
Urinanalysis, negative.
CSF: lymphs, 5 × 10^6. ℓ^{-1}.
Protein, 0.73 g. ℓ^{-1}.
Glucose, 4.8 mmol. ℓ^{-1}.
Blood lead, 0.6 μmol. ℓ^{-1}.

Questions

1. What is the most likely diagnosis?
2. Give two further useful investigations.

Case 25

A 6-year-old boy is transferred for investigation with dyspnoea and an abscess on the anterior chest wall at the right sternal border 2nd intercostal space. 1 month previously he had been admitted to a local hospital with fever, cervical lymphadenopathy, meningism, hepatosplenomegaly and right upper lobe (RUL) consolidation. Despite treatment with broad-spectrum antibiotics his condition had gradually worsened with increasing dyspnoea and finally the formation of an abscess.

He was a full-term, normal delivery, weighting 2.65 kg. There were no neonatal problems and at the age of 10 days he was adopted. He was next seen at the age of 5 months with bronchitis and loose stools. He improved on antibiotics. A sweat test was normal. At 6 months he was investigated for failure to thrive; nothing positive was found, he was placed on complan and his weight increased. At 18 months he was not walking; no specific cause was found. His bone age was approximately 6 months. At 20 months he had lymphadenitis at the angle of the right mandibular ramus. This resolved spontaneously but at 2 years he had impetigo complicated by several small abscesses on the neck; no organisms were grown and he finally responded to antibiotics. 1 year later he had mumps. At 3½ years he was found to be anaemic with hepatosplenomegaly. He was given a course of iron. At 4 years he got a chronic stye and following frequent antibiotic courses developed oral thrush. At the age of 5 years he had an anal abscess and again was noted to be small for his age. Investigations included an insulin tolerance test and jejunal biopsy. These findings were all within normal limits hence he was discharged.

Examination

Height, 1 m } both well below 3rd percentile.
Weight, 14 kg
Apyrexial.
Pulse, 88/minute.
Blood pressure, 100/65 mm Hg.
Heart sounds, soft systolic murmer left sternal edge.
Chest, dull to percussion right upper zone; bronchial breathing, right upper zone.
Abdomen: liver 4 cm enlarged; spleen, 5 cm enlarged.
Abscess: 3 × 5 cm right chest wall; fluctuant, non-tender, not

inflamed.
Rash: erythematous discrete macular rash over trunk.
Unable to walk, back painful and unable to sit without help.
Arms: normal movement, tone, power, sensation and reflexes.
Legs: both spastic, no voluntary movement on the left but 10 degree knee flexion just possible on the right. Sensation appeared intact to joint position sense and touch. Reflexes all brisk and plantars both extensor with marked bilateral ankle clonus.
Cranial nerves, intact.
Fundi, normal.

Investigations

Hb, 9.6 g. 100 ml^{-1}.
WBC, 18.9 × 10^9. ℓ^{-1}; neuts, 76%; lymphs, 23%; monos, 1%.
Platelets, 425 × 10^9. ℓ^{-1}.
IgA, 1.5 g. ℓ^{-1} (normal, 0.3–1.5 g. ℓ^{-1}).
IgG, 14.7 g. ℓ^{-1} (normal, 5–14.0 g. ℓ^{-1}).
IgM, 2.0 g. ℓ^{-1} (normal, 0.5–2.0 g. ℓ^{-1}).
Alkaline phosphatase, 448 IU. ℓ^{-1}.
AST, 24 IU. ℓ^{-1}.
ALT, 100 IU. ℓ^{-1}.
CSF: micros; 0 × 10^6 lymphs. ℓ^{-1}; 0 × 10^6 neuts. ℓ^{-1}; 165 × 10^6 RBC's. ℓ^{-1}.
Protein, 3 g. ℓ^{-1}. Culture, sterile.
Abscess fluid drained, 15 ml; culture, *Aspergillus fumigatus*.
B and T-cell numbers in peripheral blood, normal.
Phytohaemagglutinim (PHA) response within normal range.
Chest X-ray: consolidation right upper lobe; also patchy consolidation, right middle lobe.
Abdominal ultrasound: large liver and spleen, no ascites.
Bone marrow, hyperplasia of myelocytic line.
24-hour urinary vanillyl mandelic acid (VMA), not raised.

Questions

1. What is the anatomical site of the neurological lesion?.
2. What is the most likely diagnosis?
3. What four further investigations would you do?
4. What two steps in treatment would you consider?

Case 26

A 6½-year-old girl was referred urgently to Outpatients with vaginal bleeding of 4 days' duration.

The bleeding was bright red, not accompanied by any discharge and required three or four sanitary towels daily. There were no other symptoms. There was no history of recent trauma and the child denied introducing any foreign body into her vagina.

There were two older boys in the family, the mother had her menarche aged 13 years and had been sterilized after the birth of her third child.

The pregnancy had been normal, birth weight at term 3.215 kg, and there were no neonatal problems. Her development had been normal and she was of greater than average ability at school.

The parents had separated 3 years previously. The mother, aged 38 years, had remarried. The children lived with their mother and step-father, an army captain, and stayed with their father, a successful oil executive, alternate weekends.

Examination

Height, 119.8 cm (75th centile).
Weight, 21.0 kg (50th centile).
Multiple café au lait spots.
Pulse, 76/minute; sinus arrhythmia.
Heart sounds, normal.
Blood pressure, 90/55 mm Hg.
Abdomen, no masses.
Rectal examination, no masses.
No neurological abnormalities.
No secondary sexual characteristics.

Investigations

Hb, 11.3 g. 100 ml^{-1}.
WBC, $4.2 \times 10^9 . \ell^{-1}$.
Urinalysis, NAD.
Bone age, 9–9½ years.
Examination under anaesthesia (EUA): no vaginal foreign body, no vulval trauma, no abdominal masses — ovaries normal.

36

Questions

1. Give two possible diagnoses.
2. Give two further investigations to confirm the diagnosis.

Case 27

A 14-month-old boy has had a mild upper respiratory tract infection associated with occasional vomiting for the past 5 days, but for the previous 48 hours has had severe colicky abdominal pain with bloody diarrhoea and lethargy.

He was born at 36 weeks' gestation by caesarian section, weighing 2.7 kg, to a 21-year-old mother who now has another 3-month-old baby. His father is unemployed, and they live in a damp council flat. Apart from several upper respiratory infections and two episodes of otitis media, the child has been well, with his weight on the 25th centile. Developmental milestones have been normal.

Examination

Height, 72.2 cm (10th centile).
Weight, 9.3 kg (25th centile).
Pyrexial, 37.2 °C (axilla).
Pulse, 95/minute; blood pressure, 100/75 mm Hg.
Heart sounds, normal.
Chest, clear.
Pharynx, inflamed, tympanic membranes dull.
Abdomen: diffuse tenderness, no rebound tenderness.
Rectal examination, normal.
Irritable and restless.
No meningism.
No central nervous system localizing signs.

Investigations

Hb, 7.9 g. 100 ml^{-1}.
WBC: 10.2×10^9. ℓ^{-1} — polys, 80%; lymphs, 15%; monos, 4%; eosin., 1%.

Platelets, $22 \times 10^9 . \ell^{-1}$.
Prothrombin time, normal.
Partial thromboplastin time, normal.
Urea, 12 mmol. ℓ^{-1}.
Creatinine, 150 mmol. ℓ^{-1}.
Urinalysis: blood, moderate; protein, 2+.
Stool haemstest, positive.

Questions

1. What is the most likely diagnosis?
2. Give three further complications.
3. What is the pathology on microscopy?

Case 28

A 4-year-old Irish girl is admitted with a 6-week history of occasional urinary incontinence both night and day, gradually increasing in frequency. She had an intermittent pyrexia and was generally a little 'off colour' in a non-specific way. There were no other urinary symptoms and no abdominal pain. She was a full-term normal delivery with subsequent normal development and was fully continent by the age of 2½ years. Both parents were unemployed and there were three elder siblings, all in good health. They lived in a post-war prefabricated house which was so damp that water was running down the walls in two out of three bedrooms, and the family were therefore living in one bedroom and the sitting room; heating was inadequate. There was no family history of note except for the paternal grandfather, who had 'bronchitis'.

On examination her height and weight were on the 10th centile for her age and her general appearance a little unkempt.

She was kept under observation for 1 week during which time she was noted to become more withdrawn and irritable. She liked to stay in bed or sleep for an increasing length of time each day, but when got out of bed she would run around in a jerky, tremulous fashion for a short period before retiring to bed again. She became more incontinent, more difficult to rouse, and continued to have a mild pyrexia. Apart from being drowsy and irritable there were no new physical signs.

Investigations

Hb, 11.3 g. 100 ml^{-1}.
WBC: 12.6 × 10^9. ℓ^{-1} — polys, 40%; lymphs, 53%; eosins., 4%; basophils, 3%.
Urea, 5.3 mmol. ℓ^{-1}.
Electrolytes: Sodium, 135 mmol. ℓ^{-1}; potassium, 4.3 mmol. ℓ^{-1}; bicarbonate, 24 mmol. ℓ^{-1}.
Bilirubin, 17 mmol. ℓ^{-1}.
Alkaline phosphatase, 562 IU. ℓ^{-1}
AST, 12 IU. ℓ^{-1}
ALT, 17 IU. ℓ^{-1}
Blood sugar, 6.2 mmol. ℓ^{-1}.
Calcium, 2.1 mmol. ℓ^{-1}.
Urine: micro., WBC, 3 × 10^9. ℓ^{-1}; culture, 10 000 organisms/ml (both results on two specimens).
Chest X-ray — enlargement of the right hilar shadow; lung fields, clear.

Questions

1. What is the most likely diagnosis?
2. What three investigations would you do to confirm it?
3. What are two of the most common complications?
4. What two other differential diagnoses should you consider?

Case 29

An 18-month Irish child was brought to the Paediatric Ward by a Health Visitor asking for a hospital opinion. The child had been walking 3 days previously, but had suddenly refused to walk and screamed whenever his left leg touched or when the mother tried to dress or undress him.

His mother could recall no incident just prior to his refusal to walk. They lived in a 2nd-floor flat, but the only internal step led to the bathroom which always had the door shut. His mother always carried him down the external stairs.

He was the only child; his mother was 20 years old, the pregnancy had been uneventful and he was delivered at term. Birth weight, 3.685 kg. He smiled at 7 weeks, sat at 6½ months and started walking at 11 months. He could now use two-word sentences.

His father, aged 21 years, was a casual labourer with an irregular income. His mother helped to supplement this by office cleaning. They lived in a one-bedroomed, rented, private flat with shared bathroom. They were known to social services as they were often unable to pay the rent and the electricity supply had been disconnected twice. However, mother and child were reported as always being clean and well dressed.

2 months previously the parents had answered an advert in a 'Contact' magazine and they had started to frequent 'wife-swapping' parties. The husband had become involved with another woman and often spent nights with her. The wife had not been equally enamoured by the other husband and was distressed by these developments. A health visitor had then been asked to visit on a regular basis.

Examination

Height, 79.6 cm (25th centile).
Weight, 11.75 kg (50th centile).
Apyrexial.
Pulse, 98/minute; sinus arrhythmia; blood pressure, 80/45 mm Hg.
Heart sounds, normal.
Chest, abdomen and neurological systems: normal.
Tender, warm swelling of left thigh.

Investigations

Hb, 12.1 g. 100 ml^{-1}.
WBC, 5.4×10^9. ℓ^{-1}.
Blood cultures, negative.
X-ray: transverse fracture of mid-third left femur; no new bone formation, normal cortex and trabecular pattern.

On further questioning mother recalled that the child climbed onto a dining room chair, his left leg slipped through the back and the chair then fell backwards onto his leg.

Questions

1. What is the maximum age of the fracture?
2. What is the most important subsequent investigation?

Case 30

A 4-year-old Arabian child was referred to Outpatients for a second opinion on the cause of his short stature. His mother stated that he had always been small for his age, but it was only over the last 9 months that she had noticed an increasing disparity in height against his peer group. His 3-year-old brother was now taller than him.

He was born at term, by spontaneous vaginal delivery in Saudi Arabia. Birth weight unknown. He received a BCG immunization on day 2 and was discharged on day 4.

He had smiled at 7 weeks, sat at 7½ months and walked at 15 months. He could now dress and undress himself, walk up and down stairs with one foot on each stair and could obey complex commands.

3 months prior to presentation he had developed a raised, non-itchy rash behind both ears and a month ago he had begun drinking more and was waking at night to drink.

He had had one hospital admission of 3 days for gastroenteritis.

His father was in the Saudi Arabian Army, his mother had never worked.

Examination

Height, 91 cm (< 3rd centile); OFC, 48.0 cm (3rd centile).
Weight, 12.36 kg (< 3rd centile).
Father's height, 175 cm (50th centile).
Mother's height, 152 cm (3rd centile).
Pulse, 88/min; sinus arrhythmia; blood pressure, 90/60 mm Hg.
No added cardiac sounds.
Chest, clear.
Hepar, 3 cm.
Proptosis — he was unable to close his eyes completely.
Papular, non-itchy rash behind both ears.

Previous investigations

Hb, 11.9 g. 100 ml^{-1}.
WBC, 5.8 × 10^9. ℓ^{-1}.
Chest X-ray diffuse infiltration throughout.
MSU × 3, no growth.
IVP, normal.
Micturating cystogram, no reflux.

Further investigations:

Hb, 11.3 g. 100 ml^{-1}.
WBC, 6.4 × 10^9. ℓ^{-1}.
MSU, negative.
Thyroxine, 135 μmol. ℓ^{-1} (normal range 75–150 μmol. ℓ^{-1}.
TSH, 1.7 IU. ℓ^{-1} (normal range < 1–5.8 IU. ℓ^{-1}).
Serum osmolality, 296 mosmol. ℓ^{-1}.
Urine specific gravity, 1008.
Urinalysis, negative.

Questions

1. What is the diagnosis?
2. Give three further important investigations.

Case 31

A 4-month-old male infant was admitted with screaming episodes suffered for the previous 24 hours. He had been perfectly well previously, then suddenly awoke and began screaming; the episode had lasted approximately 10 minutes. He had had a further five episodes before admission. The attacks were sudden in onset, not accompanied by pallor nor with any repeated movements. There was no vomiting or diarrhoea. His mother had attempted to comfort him, but noticed that he screamed if she touched the right lower abdomen.

He was brest fed with formula-milk supplements; no solids had been introduced.

The pregnancy had been normal; delivery was via a face presentation but no resuscitative procedures were necessary.

The family lived in a modern centrally heated maisonette, the father was a policeman, and the mother worked part time in the nearby lead-smelting works. There was a healthy older sibling of 3 years.

Examination

Length, 62.9 cm (50th centile).
Weight, 6.7 kg (75th centile).
Pale irritable infant.
Pyrexial, 38.4 °C (axilla).
Pulse, 176/minute.
Respiratory and ENT systems, normal.
Abdomen, voluntary guarding generally. Right, hot tender inguinal mass — 2 × 15 cm — not transilluminable, not reducible, not fixed superficially.
Bowel sounds, normal.
Rectal examination, normal stool.
Bilateral undescended testes.

Investigations

Hb, 12.1 g. 100 ml^{-1}.
WBC, 12.5 × 10^9. ℓ^{-1} — polys, 82%; lymphs, 17%; monos, 1%.
Sodium, 141 mmol. ℓ^{-1}.
Potassium, 4.9 mmol. ℓ^{-1}.
Urea, 5.2 mmol. ℓ^{-1}.
Bag urine, WBC, 200 × 10^9. ℓ^{-1}; *E. coli* > 100 000 organisms/ml sensitive to ampicillin.
Abdominal X-ray, supine and erect —
 no fluid levels,
 no mucosal oedema.

A diagnosis of irreducible indirect inguinal hernia was returned and the child sedated and placed in gallow's traction for 36 hours. Antibiotics were started but the child demonstrated a swinging pyrexia to greater than 39 °C.

An emergency IVP showed a normal left kidney and ureter but no right kidney; ultrasound demonstrated a small right kidney and dilated ureter.

Questions

1. What is the next state of management?
2. Give three possible diagnoses.

Case 32

A female infant was born at 28 weeks' gestation, by dates, weighing 1.096 kg, the day after her mother had fallen heavily. There was no evidence of fetal distress during labour, she had a cephalic presentation and a controlled delivery. Apgar score at 1 minute, was 6 and at 5 minutes, 9. During the first hour of life she began to grunt on expiration which worsened over the next few hours. At 5 hours of life a chest X-ray showed a diffuse, uniform ground-glass appearance with air bronchograms extending beyond the border of the heart. An umbilical arterial catheter was inserted on the third attempt, and because of this antibiotics were commenced. Repeated blood gases demonstrated a falling pH and pO_2, and she was commenced on continuous positive airways pressure (CPAP) and finally on intermittent positive pressure ventilation (IPPV). A nasogastric tube was passed and aspirated two hourly, with minimal fluid recovered. On day 3 she was commenced on total parenteral nutrition. During IPPV the maximum inspiratory pressure (MIP) rate, and ambient oxygen concentration (FiO_2) were 24 cm H_2O 32/min and 0.75, respectively. On day 4 the ventilation settings were: MIPR 22/min; FiO_2 0.45; pressure, 18 cm H_2O inspiratory pressure, 4 cm H_2O expiratory pressure; inspiration: expiration (I:E) ratio 1:1.5
Blood gases: pH, 7.36; PCO_2, 5.21 kPa; PO_2, 8.5 kPa.
Bicarbonate, 21.3 mmol. ℓ^{-1}.
Base deficit, 1.8 mmol. ℓ^{-1}.
Standard bicarbonate, 22.1 mmol. ℓ^{-1}.
Standard base excess −2.2 mmol. ℓ^{-1}.

She was moving all limbs actively and was responding to being handled. She had a cyanotic episode with falling cardiac rate which did not respond to tactile stimulation, nor hand ventilation 15 minutes after the above results. She was extubated and re-intubated. The removed endotracheal tube was patent and no haemorrhage from the larynx was seen on direct vision. After re-intubation her cardiac rate remained low at between 60 and 70 beats per minute and she remained clinically cyanosed despite good air entry being heard.

Questions

1. Give two possible diagnoses.
2. Give one important investigation.

Case 33

A 10-month-old Cypriot boy was admitted with anaemia. Apart from two upper respiratory tract infections, he was well until 9 months of age, then developed a chest infection from which he made a good recovery. His GP noted that he was pale and slightly icteric.

He was born at 42 weeks' gestation by normal delivery, birth weight 3.916 kg. Developmental milestones were normal. Both parents had lived in England for some years. There was one healthy female sibling, aged 7 years.

Examination

Length, 70.2 cm (10th centile).
Weight, 8.31 kg (10th centile).
Pale.
Pulse, 100/minute — regular; blood pressure, 90/60 mm Hg.
Heart sounds, normal.
Chest, clear.
No abdominal organomegaly.
No neurological signs.

Investigations

Hb, 7.1 g. 100 ml^{-1}.
WBC; 11.0×10^9. ℓ^{-1} — lymphs, 65%; polys, 29%; eosins., 3%; monos, 3%; nucleated RBC, 3 per 100 WBC; reticulocytes, 3%.
Blood film comment: microcytes, poikilocytes and profound

hypochromia; some RBC show basophilic stippling.
Hb electrophoresis, no abnormal bands detected.
Hb F, 72%; Hb A, 25%; Hb A$_2$, 3%.
Mother: Hb F, 2%; Hb A$_2$, 3.6%.
Father: Hb F, 5.9%; Hb A$_2$, 3.9%.

Questions

1. What is the diagnosis?
2. What test can be done for antenatal diagnosis?
3. What three long-term complications may arise?

Case 34

A 6-year-old boy was referred urgently by his general practitioner for headaches and vomiting.

Three days before referral the child had been playing in the garden and had fallen about 2.4 m (8 ft) from a tree. He had been winded, but had not hit his head, and within about half an hour had been climbing the same tree. However, 2 days later he complained of headache and vomited twice. On the morning of referral he still complained of a headache and continued vomiting. He also complained that he could not see properly and his mother noticed that he had developed a squint. He was then taken to the general practitioner.

He had developed otitis media after a mild coryzal illness 2 weeks previously. He had not been taken to the general practitioner until the drum burst spontaneously and the mother noticed the discharging pus. He was treated with erythromycin and the discharge cleared in 2 days.

The child was the fifth of seven and, as far as the mother could remember, had had an unremarkable birth, birth weight unknown, and had probably been fully immunized. He had not suffered any major illness and his siblings were generally healthy also.

His parents were from Nicaragua and had been in England for 8 years. The father had been unable to gain steady employment and the mother worked as an office cleaner, the children being looked after by the eldest daughter, aged 19 years. They lived in a three-bedroomed council flat.

Examination

Height, 118.2 cm (75th centile).
Weight, 20.9 kg (50th centile).
The child was irritable and miserable but apyrexial.
Pulse, 96/min; sinus arrhythmia.
Chest clear.
Ears — both tympanic membranes normal, light reflex present, no retraction.
Throat not inflamed.
Abdominal system normal.
Nervous system: fully conscious and co-operative although irritable.
Bilateral papilloedema, pupils equal, no photophobia.
Left 6th nerve palsy.
Tone and power equal.
Reflexes, normal.
Plantars, downgoing.
Kernig's sign, negative.
Mild nuchal rigidity.
'Tripod' sign, negative.

Investigations

Hb, 12.1 g. 100 ml^{-1}.
WBC: 7.3×10^9. ℓ^{-1} — neutros, 73%; lymphs, 23%; basophils, 3%; monos, 1%.
Sodium, 131 mmol. ℓ^{-1}.
Potassium, 4.3 mmol. ℓ^{-1}.
Bicarbonate, 21 mmol. ℓ^{-1}.
Urea, 2.1 mmol. ℓ^{-1}.
Protein, 0.24 g. ℓ^{-1}.

Questions

1. Give two further important investigations.
2. What is the most likely diagnosis?
3. What is the immediate treatment?
4. Give three other causes of this problem.

Case 35

A 4-year-old boy with known IgA deficiency is admitted for investigation of failure to gain weight for 1 year, his weight now being on the 10th centile, and his height dropping from 75th to 50th centile.

He was a full-term, normal delivery, birth weight of 3 kg. He was breast fed for 1 week, then given a propietary brand of baby milk. Developmental milestones were normal. He was first admitted aged 3 months with gastroenteritis and again at 4 months with a chest infection. Investigation showed all immunoglobulin levels to be low initially, but IgG and M levels were normal by 1 year of age; IgA level remained low.

At the age of 2 years he developed constipation. This was initially treated with laxatives, enemas and an anal dilatation. For the past year, and especially recently, he has had episodes of diarrhoea and abdominal pain; the constipation has not been a problem. The stools are semi-formed, do not float, and become offensive during the episodes of diarrhoea. There is no blood or mucus. He has continued to have repeated upper respiratory tract infections including croup, not requiring admission to hospital. His appetite has been poor from the age of 1 year, he liked milk, drinking about 3 pints a day, but solids had always been a problem. His present appetite is worse than usual.

His grandfather has recently had infectious hepatitis. His sister also has IgA deficiency but with no clinical problems; his mother has hay fever. The family live in a three-bedroomed council house with garden.

Examination

Height, 101.3 cm.
Weight, 14.2 kg.
Pale, not clinically anaemic.
Pulse 84/minute; sinus arrhythmia.
Heart sounds, normal.
Chest, clear.
Pharynx, injected.
Tympanic membranes, normal.
Abdomen — not distended, no hepatosplenomegaly.
Rectal examination — no faecal loading.
No buttock wasting.

Investigations

Hb, 11.4 g. 100 ml^{-1}.
WBC: 4.7×10^9. $^{-1}$ — polys, 27%; lymphs; 67%; eosins, 1%; monos, 5%.
Platelets, normal.
Urea and electrolytes, normal.
Total protein, 76 g. ℓ^{-1}.
Albumin, 35 g. ℓ^{-1}.
Sweat sodium, 8 mmol. ℓ^{-1}.
1 h xylose after 5 g. dose, 1.69 mmol. ℓ^{-1}.
Immunoglobulins: IgA, 0.3 g. ℓ^{-1} (normal range 0.5–2.0 g. ℓ^{-1}); salivary IgA, low.
Urine, NAD.
Stool: microscopy, no ova or parasites, no fat globules; culture, no pathogens isolated.
Throat swab, no growth.

Questions

1. What is the most likely diagnosis?
2. What two further investigations would you do to establish the diagnosis?

Case 36

Adrian was delivered vaginally at term after a normal pregnancy. Breast feeding was initiated successfully; however, on day 4 he began to convulse. Lumbar puncture revelaed a Gram-negative bacterial meningitis which was treated with parenteral antibiotics for 3 weeks. During the subsequent 4 months his head circumference increased from the 25th centile to greater than the 90th centile. A CT scan demonstrated dilated ventricles so an atrioventricular shunt was inserted. The shunt was revised uneventfully at 4 years of age.

At 5 years 9 months his mother reported in Outpatients that over the past 5 weeks he had become listless, anorexic and irritable. He became tired more rapidly and was not playing as actively with his friends. She thought he had lost weight. The GP had prescribed a course of antibiotics for 10 days but without improvement.

Examination

Pale, irritable child.
Height, 106.3 cm (10th centile).
Weight, 19.4 kg (50th centile).
Temperature, 38.1 °C (oral).
Pulse, 96/min; sinus arrhythmia.
Blood pressure, 110/70 mm Hg.
Heart sounds, harsh pansystolic murmur, best heard left sternal edge.
No thrill.
Apex beat — 6th intercostal space mid-clavicular line.
Peripheral pulses, present.
Respiratory rate, 32/min.
Trachea, central.
Breath sounds, clear.
Abdomen soft — no masses palpated.
No liver swelling.
Spleen, 3 cm.
Bowel sounds, normal.
Shunt — filled and emptied rapidly.
Pupils — equal and reacting.
Fundi — no papilloedema; scattered retinal haemorrhages.
Cranial nerves, intact.
Power, co-ordination and sensation — normal.
Reflexes, normal.
Plantars, flexor.

Investigations

Hb 9.7 g. 100 ml^{-1}.
WBC: 13.6 × 10^9. ℓ^{-1} — neutros, 87%; lymphs, 9%;
Basophils 3%.
Eosinophils 1%.
Blood culture x 1 negative.
Chest X-ray — plethoric lung fields; heart — 'boot shaped'.

Questions

1 Where is the most likely anatomical position of the infective lesion?
2 What is the appropriate treatment?

Case 37

A 10-year-old boy presents with sudden onset of left-sided squint noted on waking up that morning. On closer questioning he admits to tingling of the upper lip on the left for 2-3 days but no other symptoms of note. Apart from childhood illnesses — measles, chickenpox and rubella — he has been well in the past. He had one episode of croup, aged 2 years, requiring admission to hospital. He has a sister aged 8 years. Their father works as a salesman and their mother as a secretary. They have all been well, but the maternal grandfather recently died from a stroke. At school he is average but making steady progress; he particularly likes sports and has many friends.

Examination

Height, 141 cm (75th centile).
Weight, 30.3 kg (50th centile).
Pupils, equal reaction to light; fundi, normal.
No meningism.
Minimal intention tremor on finger/nose testing on the left; no other signs of ataxia.
Marked left VIth nerve palsy.
Power, tone and sensation, equal and symmetrical.
Reflexes, normal.
General examination reveals no other abnormality.

Investigations

Hb, 13.6 g. 100 ml^{-1}.
WBC, 4.6 × 10^9. ℓ^{-1}; normal differential.
Platelets, 302 × 10^9. ℓ^{-1}.

ESR, 20 mm in first hour.
Urine analysis, NAD.
Skull X-rays, NAD.
CT scan, normal.
Audiometry, significant hearing loss on left.

He was discharged home, but readmitted 2 days later with right-sided chest pain, over the lower two or three ribs, which is dull and constant in character. He has no cough and is apyrexial. On examination there are no further physical signs; the left VIth nerve palsy is still present. The chest X-ray is clear. The pain lessened but did not disappear, so he was discharged.

He is readmitted with urinary retention 2 weeks later. He is catheterized, but requires intermittent catheterization every few days for repeated retention. He also complains intermittently of headache and difficulty in walking.

Examination reveals variable neurological signs from day to day. Sometimes he has decreased power in both legs associated with brisk reflexes, ankle clonus and extensor plantars. During several of these episodes he refused to try to walk. At other times neurological examination of his limbs is reported as normal. Cranial nerve signs remained unchanged, and general examination still reveals no abnormality.

A repeat CT scan is said to be normal.

Questions

1. What is the most likely explanation and cause of this child's problems?

Case 38

A 15-month-old West Indian child presents with failure to thrive. He was a full-term normal delivery, weighing 3.144 kg; pregnancy was normal. He was breast fed from birth and solids were introduced at 4 months of age. He had been taken regularly to a baby clinic and received all immunizations. Clinic records revealed that his weight had been around the 50th centile until about 6–9 months. Since then he had gained very little weight and when seen both height and weight were below the 3rd percentile; head circumference remained on the 50th centile. Mother had noticed swollen wrists at the age of 9 months. His general health was good, apart from several upper respiratory tract infections. His appetite was good, bowels open twice a day, and stools normal form and colour. Developmentally he had smiled at 6 weeks, sat unsupported at 10 months, was not walking yet, but could say 'Mama' and 'Dada'.

There was one sister aged 3 years, and three step-sibs who were all well. They lived in a council flat, described by the Health Visitor as 'unsatisfactory and disorganized'.

Examination

Pale.
Pulse, 92/minute; blood pressure 75/30 mm Hg.
Heart sounds, normal.
Chest, clear.
No lymphadenopathy.
No abdominal abnormality.
Obvious swelling of wrists, ankles and costochondral junctions.
No muscle wasting or oedema.

Investigations

Hb, 9.9 g. 100 ml^{-1}; Hb electrophoresis, no abnormal bands.
MCV, 65 fl.
ESR, 4 mm in first hour.
Ferritin, low.
Urea, 3.8 mmol. ℓ^{-1}.
Sodium, 140 mmol. ℓ^{-1}.
Total proteins, 60 g. ℓ^{-1}.
Potassium, 4.2 mmol. ℓ^{-1}.
Albumin, 39 g. ℓ^{-1}.
Bicarbonate, 14 mmol. ℓ^{-1}.
Calcium, 2.0 mmol. ℓ^{-1}.
Phosphate, 0.8 mmol. ℓ^{-1}.
pH: 7.38 plasma, 7.34 urine.
Alkaline phosphatase, 4800 units. ℓ^{-1}.
AST, 8 IU. ℓ^{-1}.
ALT, 15 IU. ℓ^{-1}.
Xylose absorption test, 22 mg. 100 ml^{-1} at 1 h.

Urinary amino acids, absent.
24 h urinary phosphate, 3.8 mmol. ℓ^{-1} (normal).
Acid loading test, urinary pH 5.28.
Stool microscopy, no ova or cysts seen; culture, no pathogens isolated.
3-day faecal fat excretion < 5 g daily.
MSU: microscopy, WBC 460 mm^3; culture, *E. coli* > 10^6 organism/ml.
IVP, minimal bilateral hydronephrosis and hydroureter.

Questions

1. What is the diagnosis?
2. What is the inheritance?
3. What is the treatment?

Case 39

A 5-month-old girl was referred from a district hospital for control of unprovoked temper tantrums and breath-holding attacks. The temper tantrums and breath-holding episodes had started 1 month previously. The parents were unable either to determine any provoking factors or to calm the child by any method so, in desperation, had taken her to the local hospital 2 weeks previously. The referring hospital had detected no physical or laboratory abnormalities except for two episodes of transient hypertension, thought to be secondary to her temper tantrums, and a short period of unexplained fever. Further questioning of the parents revealed that the child had been normal for the first 4 months. She was delivered vaginally at term, birth weight 2.632 kg, required no resuscitation and mother and child were discharged on day 7. She smiled at 7 weeks, was handling objects voluntarily at 3½ months, had good head control and was able to raise herself onto her elbows. At about 4 months she started drooling, became more difficult to feed and began to vomit; this was thought to be due to the recent introduction of solids. The mother also noted that even though the child was subject to crying episodes, few, if any, tears were produced.

The parents were Jewish. The father was an accountant and the mother had been an actress until the birth of their second child. The family lived in a five-bedroomed flat. The three surviving siblings were healthy; one child had died aged 14 months, no diagnosis had been established.

This infant had had two previous chest infections and was recovering from a further episode.

Examination

Weight, 6.36 kg (25th centile).
Length, 63.2 cm (50th centile).
Head circumference, 42.8 cm (50th centile).
No jaundice or clinical anaemia.
Apyrexial.
Pulse, 132/minute; blood pressure, 95/60 mm Hg.
Heart sounds, no added sounds.
No respiratory distress or recession.
Respiratory rate, 34/minute.
Right-sided basal crepitations.
Tonsils, normal.
Tympanic membranes, normal.
Tongue — smooth, drooling.
Protuberant abdomen.
Liver, 1 cm.
No splenomegaly.
Bowel sounds, normal.
Irritable.
Right-sided corneal ulceration.
Pupils, equal.
Fundi, normal.
Tone and power equal in limbs.
Spontaneous movements all limbs.
Corneal reflex, absent.
Tendon reflexes, absent.

Investigations

Hb, 11.9 g. 100 ml^{-1}.
WBC, 1.3×10^9. ℓ^{-1}.
Sodium, 139 mmol. ℓ^{-1}.
Potassium, 4.2 mmol. ℓ^{-1}.
Glucose, 5.1 mmol. ℓ^{-1}.
Bicarbonate, 26 mmol. ℓ^{-1}.

Urea, 1.9 mmol. ℓ^{-1}.
Total protein, 69 g. ℓ^{-1}.
Kaolin cephalin time (KCT)/partial thromboplastin time (PTT), within normal limits.
Liver enzymes, normal limits.
Urinalysis: pH 6; no protein, blood or reducing substances detected.
Chest X-ray, patchy atelectasis right base.

Questions

1. Give two possible diagnoses.
2. Give two further important investigations.

Case 40

A 6-year-old girl is admitted 3 weeks after the onset of chickenpox. She had not been particularly unwell on appearance of the rash, but 4 days later started vomiting. The following day she developed colicky lower abdominal pain with diarrhoea which lasted for 5 days with occasional vomiting and anorexia. Over the next 10 days she only passed two loose motions, became intermittently pyrexial and after having some difficulty in passing urine, finally developed retention.

The family are generally healthy, but her younger brother age 4 years is just developing chickenpox. In the past there has been no significant illness or operation.

Examination

Distressed child.
Pynexial, 40 °C (oral).
Pulse, 130/minute; blood pressure, 90/60 mm Hg.
Heart sounds, normal.
Chest — healing chickenpox lesions.
Abdomen soft, no tenderness; bowel sound, present.
Mass, dull to percussion, extending from public symphysis to umbilicus.
Second mass, dull to percussion, about 7 cm in diameter arose from

pelvis to right of midline behind the bladder.
Rectal examination — hard faeces marked tenderness anteriorly.
No neurological signs.

Questions

1. One important clinical procedure before further examination of patient?
2. What four important investigations would you do?
3. What is the most likely diagnosis?

Case 41

On Christmas Day a 13-year-old girl sampled her first wine; she later vomited. 2 days later she developed a coryzal illness. Initially the nasal discharge was clear, it then became purulent and she complained of a frontal headache. The headaches persisted after the resolution of the coryza. She complained of frontal pain daily but still attended school. She did not complain of visual disturbances and was not nauseated. However, after 10 days of the frontal pain she complained of numbness of the left leg and collapsed on getting up from a chair. She was conscious on admission but became comatose over the following 4 hours.

She attended the local comprehensive school and was hoping to take several 'O' levels.

She was the only child of the present marriage; the mother had a 19-year-old son by a previous marriage. The family lived in a three-bedroomed, centrally heated flat.

The patient had suffered no previous major illnesses.

Examination

Pulse, 132/minute; blood pressure, 110/65 mm Hg.
Cardiac sounds, normal.

Respiratory rate, 24/minute.
No added respiratory sounds.
Middle ear, not infected.
Semi-conscious — responded appropriately to simple commands.
Fundi — Right, gross papilloedema; left, papilloedema.
Pupils — left, reacted to light; right, ptosis and pupillary dilatation.
Cranial nerves: corneal reflex intact bilaterally; right VIth nerve palsy; no facial asymmetry.
Gag reflex intact.
Reflexes, reduced on left.
Plantars: right, downgoing; left, upgoing.

Investigations

Hb, 13.7 g. 100 ml^{-1}.
WBC, 15.3 × 10^9. ℓ^{-1}; predominantly neutrophils.
Sodium, 138 mmol. ℓ^{-1}.
Potassium, 4.2 mmol. ℓ^{-1}.
Urea, 2.3 mmol. ℓ^{-1}.
Urinalysis, negative.

A CT scan showed oedema of right cerebral hemisphere with obliteration of right ventricle, a right frontal collection of fluid and a markedly prominent falx.

The right frontal area was explored and 7 ml of pus removed from the subdural space; Gram's stain revealed Gram-positive cocci in chains and Gram-negative rods. She was commenced on parenteral broad-spectrum antibiotics.

Following surgery, she regained consciousness and the papilloedema resolved. However, she was left with a left hemiplegia and left homonymous hemianopia. She made steady progress until the third postoperative day when she became pyrexial, 40 °C (axilla), and developed left-sided fits.

Questions

1. What is the most likely origin of the infection?
2. Give two possible explanations for the extensive left-sided signs.
3. What two further investigations would you do at this stage?

Case 42

A 9-month-old child of non-consanguinous English parents is noted to have poor weight gain at the Well Baby Clinic. He has a good appetite and is on a mixed diet of tinned baby foods and cows' milk. Initially he was breast fed; complement milk formula feeds were introduced at 1 month and solids at 3 months. He passes one or two stools daily; they have always been bulky, loose and offensive. He had not been vomiting until recently when it had been in association with a paroxysmal cough.

The pregnancy was uncomplicated and he was born at term by spontaneous vaginal delivery; the birth weight was 3750 g.

He smiled at 7 weeks, rolled front to back at 6 months and sat unaided at 7 months. He now stands against the furniture and tries to crawl.

His second 'triple' vaccination was administered 2 weeks previously. The father is a policeman and the mother a librarian, before marriage. They live in police accommodation. There are two older normal siblings in the family.

Examination

A happy, alert child with no dysmorphic features.
Height, 71.2 cm (50th centile).
Weight, 7.87 kg (10th centile).
Pulse, 98/min; sinus arrhythmia; heart sounds, normal.
Respiratory rate, 40/min; slight subcostal recession.
Breath sounds, normal.
Protuberant abdomen.
No hepatosplenomegaly.
No neurological abnormalities.

Investigations

Hb, 11.1 g. 100 ml^{-1}.
WBC: 6.7×10^9. ℓ^{-1} — neutros, 69%; lymphs, 27%; monos, 4%.
Immunoglobulins: IgG, 6.3 g. ℓ^{-1} (normal range, 3–12 g. ℓ^{-1}); IgA, 0.3 g. ℓ^{-1} (normal range, 0.2–0.8 g. ℓ^{-1}); IgM, 0.6 g. ℓ^{-1} (normal range, 0.2–1.0 g. ℓ^{-1}).
Sodium, 136 mmol. ℓ^{-1}.

Potassium, 4.2 mmol. ℓ^{-1}.
Urea, 2.6 mmol. ℓ^{-1}.
Blood glucose, 4.8 mmol. ℓ^{-1}.
Serum calcium, 2.3 mmol. ℓ^{-1}.
Urinalysis, negative.
Urine culture, negative.
Chest X-ray, normal.
Bone age, 5–7 months.

Questions

1. Give three further relevant investigations.
2. Give three possible diagnoses.

Case 43

A 13-year-old girl is referred to Casualty by her general practitioner. She had been well that morning but was sent home from school complaining of headache, dizziness, difficulty in walking and finally vomiting. On questioning she said that she noticed that the letters on the blackboard had become blurred and then, later, that she staggered when she walked. The onset of symptoms had been sudden about 3 hours prior to presentation and had worsened rapidly. She had had one similar previous episode 9 months earlier.

She was not prone to headaches and no one in the family suffered from migraine. She had had no recent infective illnesses and no previous serious illnesses. She was happy at school, although rather shy and was making good academic progress.

The pregnancy had been normal and she was delivered at term, needed no resuscitation and suffered no neonatal problems. Her development was normal. She was the middle child of three. Her older brother had recently left home to join the Army; she had a younger sister.

Her father suffered from trigeminal neuralgia and was treated with carbamazepine. Her mother was a well-controlled diabetic on insulin.

Examination

On examination she was apyrexial.
Height, 150 cm (10th centile).
Weight, 42 kg (25th centile).
She had breast enlargement, but had not reached her menarche.
Cardiovascular system: pulse, 120/minute; blood pressure, 150/110 mm Hg; heart sounds, normal.
Abdominal system: low abdominal tenderness, recent perivulval bruising.
Nervous system: pupils dilated, poor response to light; fundi disc, margins clear.
She was unable to read the visual acuity chart.
Diplopia was demonstrated. She had an ataxic gait and poor hand and foot coordination.
Reflexes, brisk.
Plantars, downgoing.

Investigations

Hb, 12.1 g. 100 ml^{-1}.
WBC: 4.5×10^9. ℓ^{-1} — neutros, 72%; lymphs, 24%; monos, 3%; eosin., 1%.
Sodium, 130 mmol. ℓ^{-1}.
Potassium, 3.8 mmol. ℓ^{-1}.
Urea, 2.6 mmol. ℓ^{-1}.
Glucose, 4.1 mmol. ℓ^{-1}.
Plasma calcium, 2.1 mmol. ℓ^{-1}.
Urinalysis, negative.
Lumbar puncture: lymphs, 4×10^6. ℓ^{-1}; RBC, 200×10^6. ℓ^{-1}; glucose, 3.0 mmol. ℓ^{-1}; protein, 0.6 g. ℓ^{-1}.
Skull X-ray, normal.
The symptoms remitted 4 hours after admission with no neurological sequelae.

Discussion

1. Give one further important investigation.
2. What is the most likely diagnosis?

Case 44

A 13-year-old African girl with homozygous sickle-cell disease attended Outpatients complaining of rectal bleeding. 8 weeks previously she had developed a mild, diffuse abdominal discomfort followed shortly by diarrhoea, which had persisted. The stools were semi-solid and watery initially; but after 4 days she noticed occasional blood flecks. Each stool was now mixed with unaltered blood. Her bowel actions were not preceded or accompanied by an exacerbation of the abdominal discomfort or tenesmus, but for the last few days she had noted soiling on her underwear. She was unaware of being incontinent. She had lost sufficient weight to notice that her clothes were now fitting loosely.

She had not been abroad during the past year, but an uncle from Nigeria had been staying with the family for the last 4 months. No other member of the family was suffering from diarrhoea.

Sickle-cell disease had been diagnosed at 11 months of age and she had been maintained on daily folic acid supplements. She had had only a few sickle 'crises'; her last admission had been 2 years previously.

She was one of seven children, one other of whom had sickle-cell disease. Both parents were unemployed and the family lived in a damp, three-bedroomed council maisonette.

Examination

Height, 143.1 cm (3rd centile).
Weight, 28.9 kg (< 3rd centile).
Conjunctivae, pale.
Pulse, 94/minute; blood pressure, 110/60 mm Hg.
Cardiac sounds: soft, short mid-systolic murmur, maximal at left sternal edge.
Tender mass in right iliac fossa, approximately 5 × 8 cm.
No hepatosplenomegaly.

Investigations

Hb, 3 months previously 8.6 g. 100 ml^{-1}; now 8.3 g. 100 ml^{-1}.
Reticulocyte count, 7%.
Sodium, 136 mmol. ℓ^{-1}.
Potassium, 4.1 mmol. ℓ^{-1}.

Bicarbonate, 24 mmol. ℓ^{-1}.
Urea, 2.7 mmol. ℓ^{-1}.

Questions

1. Give two possible diagnoses.
2. Give two further helpful investigations to establish the diagnosis.

Case 45

A 19-month-old girl is admitted after a febrile convulsion. She had had a cough for 3 days and been pyrexial for 8 hours. Mother found her lying in a pool of vomit in bed, blue with her eyes rolled upwards.

She had been born by elective caesarian section at term, birth weight 3.57 kg. She was breast fed for 5 months, had no problems and normal developmental milestones. Over the previous winter she had had three attacks of 'wheezy bronchitis' but no previous fits. The maternal grandfather has asthma.

On examination her temperature was 41 °C, she was cyanosed and twitching. Cervical lymphadenopathy was marked and respiratory rate 48/min. The throat was inflamed with no exudate and both tympanic membranes were dull. The chest was hyperinflated, breath sounds equal in right and left lungs with crepitations in the left anterior–lateral area. Her pulse was 180/min, her heart sounds normal. There was no hepatosplenomegaly or other positive abdominal signs and no meningism.

Investigations

Hb, 13.1 g. 100 ml^{-1}.
WBC: 17.8 × 10^9. ℓ^{-1}. — polys, 79%; lymphs, 20%.
Platelets, normal.
CSF: micros., 30 × 10^6. ℓ^{-1} RBC, no WBC; culture, no growth.
Blood culture, no growth.
Throat swab, no growth.
Mantoux test, negative.

Chest X-ray, linear shadowing, left mid-zone.

She was treated with ampicillin and flucloxacillin intravenously, but on changing to oral antibiotics 2 days later she became irritable and pyrexial. Repeat lumbar puncture was traumatic.

CSF: micros., RBC, $2378 \times 10^6 . \ell^{-1}$; WBC, $91 \times 10^6 . \ell^{-1}$; lymphs, $28 \times 10^6 . \ell^{-1}$.

Gram's stain, no organisms seen.

Chloramphenicol was added to the medication. The temperature settled and her general condition improved.

3 days later she was noted to have markedly decreased chest movements on the left, the percussion note was hyper-resonant on the left and breath sounds reduced. The following day a 'brassy' cough developed; chest signs were unchanged. Repeat chest X-ray showed hyperinflation of the left lung.

Questions

1. What is the diagnosis?
2. What is the treatment?

Case 46

A 10-year-old boy is referred to Outpatients from a country residential home with a provisional diagnosis of retinoblastoma. He had complained of poor vision in the right eye and was noted to have absence of the red reflex and a white raised plaque arising from the temporal side of the retina. No systemic abnormalities were noted.

In Outpatients the boy complained of no symptoms other than of visual loss. His housemother stated that he was generally healthy, had a good appetite and did not become unduly tired on physical exertion. He was of average intelligence with an Intelligence Quotient (IQ) of 90. No pets were allowed in the Children's Home.

He had been taken into care 2 years previously following the prosecution of his parents for child abuse, at which time a small white fibrotic lesion was noted in the temporal area of the right retina during his admission examination. He was the third of five children; two others were also in care. The family lived in a terraced house which faced an area of wasteland on which the children played.

Examination

Height, 142 cm (75th centile).
Weight, 31 kg (75th centile).
Apyrexial, no skin rashes.
Cardiovascular and respiratory systems normal; no hepatosplenomegaly; no abdominal masses. Small, firm inguinal lymph nodes were palpable bilaterally.
Pupils equal and reacting to light, no proptosis.
Fundi: left, normal; right, large white raised irregular plaque.
Visual fields, large scotoma in right nasal field.
Reflexes, normal.
Plantars, downgoing.

Investigations

Hb, 12.5 mg. 100 ml^{-1}.
WBC: $16.7 \times 10^9. \ell^{-1}$ — neutros, 43%; lymphs, 10%; eosin., 35%; monos, 3%.
Skull and chest X-ray, normal.
Urinalysis, normal.

Questions

1. Give one further important investigation.
2. What is the most likely diagnosis?

Case 47

An 18-month-old boy was admitted from the Middle East with 'bone disease'. He was a full-term, normal delivery weighing approximately 3 kg. He appeared normal at birth but had failed to thrive since. On admission he weighed 6.8 kg, height was 70 cm (well below 3rd centile) and head circumference on the 50th centile. He had had constipation for some weeks and vomiting for the last 3 days.

Developmental milestones were not known, but he had never been able to walk. His mother was aged 35 and father aged 48; they were first cousins. Six siblings aged 12–17 were alive and well, but four others had all died of 'vomiting' aged less than 1 year.

On examination he was an extremely wasted child, dehydrated with gross rickets. Respiratory rate, 40/min but the chest was clear and heart sounds normal.

The abdomen was generally distended, liver edge just palpable, bowel sounds absent, and rectal examination revealed hard, formed stool.

In the CNS he was markedly apathetic and lethargic with reduced tone but no focal signs.

Investigations

Hb, 13.3 g. 100 ml^{-1}.
WBC: 12.0×10^9. ℓ^{-1} — polys, 71% with left shift.
Urea, 7.2 mmol. ℓ^{-1}.
Sodium, 126 mmol. ℓ^{-1}.
Potassium, 1.4 mmol. ℓ^{-1}.
Bicarbonate, 11 mmol. ℓ^{-1}.
Blood sugar, 3.5 mmol. ℓ^{-1}.
Phosphate, 0.94 mmol. ℓ^{-1}.
Calcium, 2.1 mmol. ℓ^{-1}.
Alkaline phosphatase, 1560 IU. ℓ^{-1}.
Chest X-ray: lung fields clear; heart normal. Extensive loss of bone trabeculae in the ribs and a number of fractures are present.
Limb X-rays: gross demineralization of all bones. Appearance consistent with rickets possibly associated with vitamin D deficiency.
Urine analysis, pH 6.0; protein, +; glucose, trace.

Questions

1. What is the diagnosis?
2. What is the most likely cause?
3. What three further investigations would you do to confirm the diagnosis?
4. What are the three most important factors in long-term management of this child?
5. Name two other causes of this syndrome?

Case 48

A 14-year-old boy was referred to a child guidance clinic for assessment of episodes of uncontrollable aggression. He had been an affectionate and placid child until he was 8 years old when his parents separated and his father refused to see the children. He gradually became withdrawn and had aggressive outbursts when confronted by his mother over any misdemeanour. However, over the past 13 months some episodes had become unpredictable and were usually associated with abdominal pain. The general practitioner initially diagnosed abdominal migraine and prescribed analgesics and laxatives but to no effect; it was then suggested that the diagnosis was temporal lobe epilepsy. An EEG was normal and a trial of carbamazepine failed to relieve the attacks. The child was then referred to child guidance. He was seen at the initial interview with his mother and 11-year-old sister, where it was felt that individual psychotherapy was appropriate.

The father was a lock-keeper and the family lived in a cottage by the lock. Father and son had spent a great deal of time together, either on their own boat or fishing. However, he was made redundant and the family had to move to the local town, where the mother gained employment as a domestic cleaning lady.

Thereafter the relationship between husband and wife deteriorated and he eventually left. The child interpreted this as the mother forcing the father to go because he did not have a job, and refusing access to the children. He, therefore, reacted aggressively towards correction and expressed a desire to kill his mother. He was frank about these emotions but was puzzled about, and scared of, his unpredictable outbursts.

During one such aggressive episode he became violent and the police were called, who took him to the local police station where he was seen by a police surgeon and referred to the Accident and Emergency Department.

Examination

Aggressive, uncooperative child.
Height, 163.9 cm (75th centile).
Weight, 48.9 kg (50th centile).
Pyrexial, 38.4 °C.
No clinical jaundice or anaemia.
Pulse, 112 beats/min; blood pressure, 140/90 mm Hg.

Soft, mid-systolic murmur in the pulmonary area varied with position.
No hepatosplenomegaly.
Left otitis media.
Neurological system — refused to answer questions.
Pupils, reacted to light.
Fundi, normal.
Loss of deep tendon reflexes; plantars, downgoing.
Pigmented areas on forearms, back of hands and malar region of the face.
Evidence of secondary sexual development: enlargement of penis and testes, scanty pubic hair; his voice had broken.

Investigations

Hb, 14.1 g. 100 ml^{-1}.
WBC, 15.6 × 10^9. ℓ^{-1}.
Sodium, 128 mmol. ℓ^{-1}.
Potassium, 4.6 mmol. ℓ^{-1}.
Glucose, 6.7 mmol. ℓ^{-1}.
Urea, 7.4 mmol. ℓ^{-1}.

Questions

1. What is the most likely diagnosis?
2. What is the inheritance of the disease?

Case 49

A 11-week-old male infant was brought to Casualty with a history of lethargy, poor feeding and weight loss. He was a full-term, normal delivery, birth weight 3.1 kg, and had had no perinatal problems. He had been seen in Casualty 4 weeks previously with vomiting and had been treated with clear fluids. A follow-up outpatient appointment was made but he never attended. Apparently he had gradually become less interested in his feeds, eventually taking approximately 2 fl oz (57 cm^3) per feed 3–4 times a day. There had been occasional vomits but no diarrhoea. Various milks had been tried with little success.

The parents were not married. His mother was English, aged 22 years, and had married a Thai man in order for him to gain entry to the UK. She was co-habiting with another Thai man, the father of the child, who was due to return to Thailand in the near future.

On examination the baby was marasmic, weighing 2.9 kg. He was miserable with an anxious look and ammoniacal nappy rash, but no other abnormality. He was admitted to hospital and given regular feeds of a proprietary baby milk at 150 ml.kg^{-1} daily. Initially he took feeds eagerly and gained weight, but after 2 days became disinterested. Tube feeding resulted in a marked increase in vomiting but no diarrhoea.

Investigations

Hb, 11.4 g. 100 ml^{-1}.
WBC; 14.2 × 10^9. ℓ^{-1} — normal differential; film, normal.
Urea, 2.0 mmol. ℓ^{-1}.
Sodium, 137 mmol. ℓ^{-1}.
Potassium, 3.8 mmol. ℓ^{-1}.
Bicarbonate, 30 mmol. ℓ^{-1}.
Urine microscopy and culture, normal.
Stool culture, no pathogens.
Urine: reducing substances, negative; 24-hour VMA excretion, normal.
Chest X-ray, normal.

Questions

1. Give three possible diagnoses in order of priority.
2. Give three investigations that you would carry out immediately to help prove the most likely diagnosis.

Case 50

A 15-year-old primigravida schoolgirl was admitted in established labour. The pregnancy had been concealed until late and she had not attended any antenatal clinics. Her periods had been irregular before pregnancy, but the head was engaged and the fundal height was compatible with a term pregnancy. Labour proceeded uneventfully and she was delivered of a normal female infant. Apgar scores were 7 at 1 minute and 9 at 5 minutes. Birth weight, 3.510 kg. Breast feeding was attempted unsuccessfully and bottle feeding was commenced on day 4. On day 3 the baby was noticed to be jaundiced, serum bilirubin 186 μmol. ℓ^{-1}; this rose to 225 μmol. ℓ^{-1} the following day and she was treated effectively with intermittent phototheraphy for 3 days. However, the jaundice recurred after the cessation of treatment and it was noticed that there had been poor weight gain. She had lost 196 g in the first 2 days and subsequently had gained only 15 g. Phototherapy was recommenced and she had supplementary feeds via an indwelling nasogastric tube. On day 10 she was still jaundiced and had now developed non-bloody diarrhoea and vomiting.

Examination

Weight, 3.415 kg.
Clinically jaundiced.
Pulse, 138/min; blood pressure, 65/40 mm Hg.
Heart sounds, normal.
Hepar, 3.5 cm.
No splenomegaly.
Lethargic but irritable on handling.
Tone, poor.

Investigations

Hb, 14.7 g. 100 ml^{-1}.
WBC, 11.6 $\times$ 10^9. ℓ^{-1}.
Glucose, 1.9 mmol. ℓ^{-1}.
Bilirubin, 186 μmol. ℓ^{-1}.
PTT/KCCT, prolonged.
Blood gases: pH, 7.29; pCO$_2$, 4.2 KPa; pO$_2$, 11.7 KPa; bicarbonate, 21.3 mmol; base excess, -6.7 mmol. ℓ^{-1}; standard bicarbonate, 18 mmol. ℓ^{-1}; standard base excess, -7.0 mmol. ℓ^{-1}.
Lumbar puncture: lymphocyte 3 $\times$ 10^6. ℓ^{-1}; protein, 0.4 g. ℓ^{-1}; glucose, 1.6 mmol. ℓ^{-1}.
Antibodies to: Toxoplasma, 1:8; Cytomegalovirus, 1:8; Rubella, 1:16; Herpes, 1:8.
Urinalysis, Clinitest positive.
Stool reducing substances, negative.

Questions

1. Give two possible diagnoses.
2. Give three further important investigations.

Case 51

A 10-year-old boy who has completed 2½ years of treatment for common ALL on a UKALL regimen without relapse and been off treatment for 7 months presents with a mild pyrexia and generalized pains. 3 weeks previously he had had a heavy cold with the rest of his family and following this he had gradually developed swelling of his ankles and elbows. 5 days before he had been reluctant to go to school in the morning, walked slowly and refused to put on his coat despite the cold weather. After 2 days of similar behaviour his mother realized that he could not extend his elbows. He had lost 4 kg in weight even though his appetite was fair.

His father works as a dental technician and his mother as a barmaid. There is a brother aged 16 years. All were in good health.

Examination

Height, 136.5 cm (50th centile).
Weight, 26.5 kg (25th centile).
Pyrexial, 37.8 °C (oral).
Pulse, 97/minute; sinus arrhythmia.
Blood pressure, 110/70 mm Hg.
Heart sounds, normal.
Chest, clear.
Abdomen, normal.
Mouth, no discoloration.
Tongue, marginal atrophy.
Cranial nerves, unable to protrude tongue fully.
Erythematous rash on upper eyelids, shoulders, upper chest and front of thighs.
Pitting oedema of both feet and ankles to mid-calf level and around elbows.
Generalized muscle wasting with fasciculation, marked over upper limb girdle.

Movement in all joints painful.
Neck: limited extension, rotation; flexion normal.
Elbows, 110 degree fixed flexion.
Shoulder, 90 degree abduction.
Fingers — difficulty with fine movements.
Hips, flexion 45 degrees.
Ankles — painless normal movement.

Investigations

Hb, 13.7 g. 100 ml^{-1}.
ESR, 4 mm in first hour.
WBC: 12.5×10^9. ℓ^{-1} — polys, 80%; lymphs, 12%; monos, 8%.
Platelets, 251×10^9. ℓ^{-1}.
Urea, 6.1 mmol. ℓ^{-1}.
Calcium, 2.25 mmol. ℓ^{-1}.
Sodium, 136 mmol. ℓ^{-1}.
Total protein, 66 g. ℓ^{-1}.
Potassium, 4.2 mmol. ℓ^{-1}.
Alkaline phosphatase, 319 IU.
X-rays, elbow and ankles, NAD.
Chest X-ray, no abnormality.
Immunoglobulins: IgG, IgA, IgM, normal.
Urinalysis, NAD.

Questions

1. What are three differential diagnoses in order of priority?
2. What three investigations would you do immediately?
3. What three other physical signs might one expect to see or develop?

Case 52

An 8-year-old girl is referred to Outpatients with a 4-month history of headaches and vomiting. She had been treated by her general practitioner with analgesics and antiemetics but these had afforded only temporary relief.

The headaches were frontal, not throbbing and were usually present on awakening but tended to improve during the day. The vomiting was variable but was not associated with any foodstuffs nor accompanied by nausea. These episodes occurred on any day and did not resolve at the weekends or during school holidays. There was no aura and she was not drowsy or disorientated either during or after the episode. She had never suffered a convulsion and there was no family history of fits.

The pregnancy had been normal and there were no problems in the neonatal or infantile periods. She sat at 6 months, walked at 14 months and was reported as average in school.

The family lived in an old terraced house in an industrial area. The house had recently been replumbed and redecorated. Her father was a 46-year-old steel worker and her mother, aged 39 years, worked part-time in a factory canteen. There were three healthy siblings aged 12 years, 9 years and 5 years.

Examination

Height, 126.4 cm (75th centile).
Weight, 28.7 kg (90th centile).
Apyrexial.
Pulse, 68/min; sinus arrhythmia; blood pressure, 125/85 mm Hg.
Peripheral pulses, normal.
No added heart sounds.
ENT: healthy tympanic membranes, positive light reflexes.
No abdominal masses.
Pupils: equal and reacting to light.
Fundi: discs pink, veins engorged.
No nystagmus.
Cranial nerves, no abnormality.
Power, normal in all limbs.
Gait: unsteady, wide based.
Standing and sitting: truncal ataxia.
Co-ordination: upper limbs good; lower limbs, poor.
Heel–shin test, normal; sensation, normal.
Reflexes: normal plantars, extensor.

Investigations

Hb, 14.1 g. 100 ml^{-1}.
WBC, 6.8×10^9. ℓ^{-1}.

Sodium, 139 mmol. ℓ^{-1}.
Potassium, 4.3 mmol. ℓ^{-1}.
Urea, 2.1 mmol. ℓ^{-1}.
Protoporphyrins, 24 ng. dl^{-1} (normal range < 50 ng. dl^{-1}).
ECG Axis, + 85 degrees.
Skull X-ray: erosion of the posterior clinoid process.

Questions

1. What is the most likely diagnosis?
2. Give one further important investigation.

Case 53

An 8-year-old boy with Down's syndrome was admitted for revision of the distal catheter of his atrioventricular Spitz–Holter valve. The valve had been inserted at 10 weeks of age and had required revision once only at 3 years of age.

He was born at 39 weeks' gestation by dates, birth weight 2.377 kg, from a 42-year-old mother after a normal pregnancy. The diagnosis of trisomy 21 was made clinically at birth and confirmed on chromosome analysis. On the second day of life he developed mild jaundice and a diffuse but discrete, erythematous maculopapular rash. The rash cleared within the first week, the jaundice within the first 3 weeks.

Both parents rejected him initially but, after counselling, they accepted him home aged 17 days.

He was seen regularly in Outpatients where it was noticed that his head circumference was increasing rapidly. Air ventriculography at 10 weeks demonstrated dilated lateral ventricles and an atrioventricular valve was inserted.

He was able to walk unaided but was unable to help in dressing or undressing. He was unable to talk but would obey simple commands. He attended a school for the severely educationally subnormal.

He was the third child; the other siblings were 18 and 20 years old and both had left home. The family now lived in a two-bedroomed flat over their fish and chip shop.

Examination

Height, 113.3 cm (3rd centile).
Weight, 21.7 kg (10th centile).
Many stigmata of trisomy 21.
Pulse, 98/min.
Heart sounds: apex, short midsystolic murmur, long diastolic murmur; base, ejection systolic murmur.
Breath sounds, normal.
No hepatosplenomegaly.
Responded to simple commands, e.g. shut the door.
Pupils: equal and reactive to light; no cataracts.
Fundi: bilateral diffuse choroidoretinitis.
Reflexes, normal.
Plantars, downgoing.

Investigations

ECG: sinus rhythm, left axis deviation.

Questions

1. Give one further important investigation.
2. Give two possible diagnoses.

Case 54

A 7½-year-old boy is referred to Outpatients for investigation of recurrent abdominal pain over the last 18 months. The attacks occurred at 4-monthly intervals initially, but more recently every 4–6 weeks, on occasion necessitating sending the boy home from school. His GP had never found any positive physical signs but treated him for a possible urinary tract infection with antibiotics.

The episodes of pain would start on the left side of the abdomen, any time of the day or night, and gradually become generalized. At the same time he became pyrexial, his temperature ranging up to 39 °C, flushed, agitated and nauseated with copious vomiting but no diarrhoea. There were no urinary symptoms. At these times he liked to go to bed and after approximately 24 hours the pain would suddenly resolve and within 1 hour he would be back to his normal self.

He was a full-term normal delivery with no problems apart from being a 'sickly' baby. He is the only natural child of the parents, who are both English. His mother is a registered child-minder. Another boy, 16 months younger, with asthma and eczema, has been living with the family for about 3 years on long-term fostering. The father works as a head porter in a block of flats. Family relationships are said to be good and school work satisfactory.

On examination there were no abnormal physical signs.

Investigations

FBC, normal.
ESR, 3 mm in first hour.
MSU: micros, less than 3×10^9 WBC. ℓ^{-1}; culture, no significant growth.
Urinalysis, negative.
Urine porphobilinogen, normal.

Questions

1. What two further points in the history would you like to know?
2. What two steps would you like to take to help you make a diagnosis?

Case 55

A 3½-year-old boy was seen frequently by his general practitioner for recurrent chest infections. He had been admitted to hospital at 7 months of age with a pertussis infection and then again at 11 months with bronchiolitis. Since then he had had several chest infections, usually following an upper respiratory tract infection. Each time he had been treated with antibiotics by his GP, the symptoms resolving in the following 2–3 weeks. However, even when clinically well he still had coughing episodes, especially in the morning. He was, therefore, referred to Outpatients for specialist advice.

Further questioning revealed that he had always had a good appetite but gained weight slowly, he had two or three bowel actions daily and there was no undue vomiting. He was an active child and played happily with friends and at nursery school, but frequently he would have a coughing burst after exertion. This coughing worsened during his chest infections and on the rare occasions when he was persuaded to expectorate mucopus, intermittently streaked with blood, was produced.

He was the only child of older parents. His father was aged 53 years and mother 43 years; both were university lecturers and they lived in a modern university flat.

The pregnancy had been complicated by maternal toxaemia and delivery was induced at 37 weeks' gestation. The infant weighed 2.650 kg at birth. He was of normal intelligence, he walked at 13 months and was now obeying commands and dressing and undressing himself with help.

Examination

Apyrexial, not cyanosed, mild clubbing of fingers.
Pulse, 96/minute.
Apex beat, 5th intercostal space, 1 cm lateral to mid-clavicular line.
Heart sounds, normal.
Peripheral pulses, present.
Respiratory rate, 28/minute.
No recession.
Percussion normal.
Bilateral basal crepitations.
Hepar, 1 cm.
No spleen palpable.
Bowel sounds, normal.
Irritable child but not neurological abnormalities.

Investigations

Weight, 11.83 kg.
Height, 91 cm.
Hb, 14.3 g. 100 ml^{-1}.
WBC: 9.7×10^9. ℓ^{-1} — neutros, 78%; lymphs, 19%; basophils, 1%; monos, 2%.
Sodium, 130 mmol. ℓ^{-1}.

Potassium, 3.6 mmol. ℓ^{-1}.
Calcium, 2.01 mmol. ℓ^{-1}.
Glucose, 4.6 mmol. ℓ^{-1}.
Total protein, 64 g. ℓ^{-1}.
Albumin, 39 g. ℓ^{-1}.
Urea, 1.9 mmol. ℓ^{-1}.
Sputum, mixed flora.
Urinalysis: pH 6; nil else detected.
ECG, right-sided strain pattern.

Questions

1. Give three further useful investigations.
2. Give two important lines of treatment.

Case 56

An 8-year-old boy is admitted via Casualty for the third time in 3 months with similar symptoms of severe pain at the tip of the penis on micturition, frequency and lower abdominal pain. He had been enuretic all his life. He had first developed these symptoms 17 months earlier. Nothing was found on examination and investigation showed no urinary tract infection and a normal IVP. He improved spontaneously but had a similar episode lasting 5 weeks, 6 months later.

He was admitted for investigation 14 months after the initial episode. Expression cystogram done under general anaesthetic was normal, and he was left catheterized for 24 hours because of difficulty in passing the cystoscope. On catheter removal he continued to have severe difficulty in passing urine and requiring another general anaesthetic for insertion of a suprapubic catheter.

He gradually improved. Erythromycin was given for treatment of urethritis but no cause was found. 2 weeks after admission he developed vomiting and upper abdominal pain, there was nothing to find on examination and he was discharged home 5 days later, still vomiting occasionally.

He was readmitted 1 week later and had another general

anaesthetic for cystourethroscopy. Urethral stricture was found with a proximally dilated urethra and a hypertrophied bladder. A suprapubic catheter was inserted and erythromycin re-started. Two further urethral dilatations were done during the next 10 days, both under general anaesthetic. Prior to the second, 'odd' behaviour was noted, in that he was screaming inappropriately, soiling deliberately and biting the thermometer. He continued to be 'difficult' on the ward and 1 week later, when ready to go home, he started vomiting, screaming and complaining of substernal pain and headache. Mother did not want her son to have psychiatric help and he was discharged still on erythromycin.

On his third admission, 5 weeks later, he developed acute urinary retention. Expression cystogram under general anaesthetic revealed a markedly dilated urethra except for the final 1 cm which was severely constricted. An extensive meatotmy was done and suprapubic catheter inserted. Nausea, vomiting, abdominal pain and mild drowsiness developed 5 days after the operation.

Examination

Height, 126.5 cm (50th centile).
Weight, 21.0 kg (10th centile).
Pyrexial, 37.4 °C (oral).
Fully conscious and orientated.
Mild jaundice.
Pulse, 90/minute, regular; blood pressure, 100/70 mm Hg.
Heart sounds, normal.
Chest, clear.
Fauces, normal.
No lymphadenopathy.
Abdomen: liver, tipped, non-tender; spleen, not palpable; no ascites.
No tremor or flap.
No focal neurological signs.

Investigations

Hb, 11.8 g. 100 ml^{-1}.
WBC: 10.6×10^9. ℓ^{-1} — polys, 54%; lymphs, 38%; eosin., 1%; monos, 8%.
Film: target cells, some active lymphocytes.
Platelets, 218×10^9. ℓ^{-1}.
Monospot, negative.

Prothrombin time, 59 s; control, 14 s.
Kaolin cephalin clotting time (KCCT) 98 s; control, 35 s.

Table 1
Initial results and results taken 2 weeks later. Figures in parentheses show normal ranges

Test	Initial	2 weeks later
Total bilirubin (mmol. ℓ^{-1})	80	480
Conjugated bilirubin (mmol. ℓ^{-1})	40	270
Alkaline phosphatase (IU. ℓ^{-1})	685	995
ALT (IU. ℓ^{-1})	1379	170
AST (IU. ℓ^{-1})	1110	385
Albumin (g. ℓ^{-1})	33	26
IgG	7.5 (5–14)	12.7
IgA	1.7 (0.5–2.5)	2.2
IgM	8.0 (0.5–2.0)	3.1

Anti-hepatitis A virus IgM, negative.
Hepatitis B surface antigen, negative.
CMV IgM, negative.
Epstein–Barr virus (EBV) IgM, negative.
Herpes simplex IgM, negative.
MSU, NAD.
Stools: no ova or cysts; no pathogens grown.
Autoantibodies: smooth muscle, 1+; liver–kidney microsomes, strongly positive; all others, negative.
Ammonia, 139 μmol. ℓ^{-1} (normal < 40).

Questions

1. What three differential diagnoses would you consider most likely?
2. What four important investigations would you do?
3. What three necessary steps in treatment would you start?

Case 57

A 3-year-old child attended Outpatients for cyanotic episodes. The first episode had been 7 months previously. The child had had an upper respiratory tract infection and on going to sleep she began to snore and then became cyanosed. The episode was aborted when the mother awoke the child and sat her upright. The next episode was several weeks later. The episode again occurred as the child was going to sleep and aborted as before. The attacks became more frequent, especially if associated with an upper respiratory tract infection, all occurring on falling asleep and all easily aborted. The child had never developed stridor but she was a mouth-breather and had had no cyanotic episodes whilst awake.

She was a term infant, born vaginally, birth weight 3.24 kg. She was the third child. The father, aged 41 years, was a miner and the mother, aged 36 years, was a food packer at the local factory. The family lived in a two-bedroomed terraced house with open-coal fires.

Examination

Apyrexial.
Height, 90.7 cm (25th centile).
Weight, 13.2 kg (25th centile).
Pulse, 90/minute; blood pressure, 80/55 mm Hg.
Parasternal heave.
Apex beat, mid-clavicular line, 5th interspace; second sound — wide-splitting — moving with respiration.
No murmurs.
Peripheral pulses, normal.
Mouth breathing.
No added respiratory sounds.
No abdominal or neurological abnormalities.

Investigations

Hb, 12.1 g. 100 ml^{-1}.
WBC, 5.9×10^9. ℓ^{-1}.
Chest X-ray — enlarged cardiac shadow.
ECG: axis + 90 degrees; right ventricular hypertrophy.

Table 1
Cardiac catheter studies

Pressures (mm Hg)	Oxygen saturation (%)
Superior vena cava	69
Right atrium, m = 6	67
Right ventricle, 110/6	66
Pulmonary artery, 105/45	66
Pulmonary wedge pressure, 5	

Questions

1. What is the most likely aetiology of her cardiovascular problems?

Case 58

A 7-year-old girl presents with a 3-month history of pain in the shoulders, elbows, hips and knees. Her parents feel that she is not as active as she used to be; in particular she has not been able to walk as far as before, one of the family's favourite pursuits being hiking. At the end of the day she feels weak but is not anxious to go upstairs to bed. Apart from this her general health has been good with no intercurrent infections and no previous history of note. She has a brother and sister, both of whom are older and who are well. There has been no recent illness in the family.

She was seen by her general practitioner, who could find no abnormal clinical signs and prescribed aspirin. The pain improved but she appeared to get weaker.

On examination she was apyrexial with no rash or lymphadenopathy. General examination of heart, chest and abdomen and central nervous system was normal apart from slightly reduced tendon reflexes.

Musculoskeletal examination revealed no abnormality in the joints and non-tender muscles. The facial expression was normal but neck extension and shoulder adduction were weak, and there was slight winging of both scapulae. She had a waddling gait, difficulty in getting off the floor without assistance and weakness of the gluteal muscles. Other muscles appeared normal.

Investigations

Hb, 12 g. 100 ml^{-1}.
WBC: $6.3 \times 10^9 . \ell^{-1}$ — polys, 46%; lymphs, 49%; eosins., 3%; basophils, 2%.
Platelets, $320 \times 10^9 . \ell^{-1}$.
Paul–Bunnell test, negative.
ESR, 15 mm in first hour.
AST, normal.

ALT, normal.
Alkaline phosphatase, 320 units.
Antistreptolysin 'O' titre (ASOT) < 60 units.
Antinuclear factor (ANF), negative.
Rheumatoid factor (RF) — Negative.
Throat swab: β-haemolytic streptococci, group B.
Nose swab, *Staphylococcus aureus*.

Questions

1. What is the most likely diagnosis?
2. What three investigations would you carry out to aid diagnosis?

Case 59

A 14-year-old boy was admitted with a chest infection and right-sided heart failure. He suffered from chronic granulomatous disease and had had recurrent chest infections. These had produced sufficient lung damage to cause incipient cor pulmonale. He was maintained on regular digoxin and also salbutamol, which improved his peak flow.

He had had a bone-marrow transplant 3 years previously from a related donor. The graft had taken initially but then gradually failed as his own marrow regenerated. No further transplants had been attempted.

He had developed a cough 4 days prior to this admission. He had been commenced on co-trimoxazole immediately, but he had gradually worsened and was admitted with a productive cough and right-sided failure.

He had been adopted at the age of 5 years. His adoptive parents, who had one son of their own, had been fully conversant with his condition at the time of adoption.

He attended the local grammar school, but had additional private tuition to minimize the effect of repeated hospital admissions.

Examination

Height, 140.2 cm (< 3rd centile).
Weight, 32.7 kg (< 3rd centile).

Centrally cyanosed.
Pulse, 112/min; blood pressure, 110/70 mm Hg.
Parasternal heave.
Mid-systolic ejection murmur, maximal in the pulmonary area.
Hyperinflated chest with increased anteroposterior diameter — poor respiratory excursion — accessory respiratory muscles used.
Bilateral scattered crepitations and rhonchi.
Smooth, non-tender hepatomegaly of 2 cm.
Deformity of left upper arm and right femur from episodes of osteomyelitis.

Investigations

Hb, 14.6 g. 100 ml^{-1}.
WBC: 15.7 × 10^9. ℓ^{-1} — neutros, 73%; lymphs, 24%; monos, 2%; eosins., 1%.
pH 7.36.
P_{O_2}, 7.5 kPa.
P_{CO_2}, 6.9 kPa.
Bicarbonate, 31 mmol. ℓ^{-1}.
Base excess, 5 mmol. ℓ^{-1}.

He was given oxygen by mask and commenced on carbenicillin and tobramycin. Theophylline was added in view of worsened wheezing. He improved gradually and after 48 hours was no longer cyanosed; however, he was noted to have coupling beats.

Questions

1. What are the two most important investigations?

Case 60

A 14-month-old Bangladeshi boy was referred with a 1-month history of 'eye problems'. The father was a very poor historian, and mother spoke no English. The eyes were said to be flitting from side to side. His appetite had decreased over the previous 6 months but there were no other symptoms of note.

He was a full term, normal delivery weighing 2.466 kg with no neonatal problems, the first child of unrelated parents. He had been breast fed for 8 months, then his mother had become pregnant again, so he was weaned on to a proprietary milk, together with some solid food such as rice. He had occasional vomits but no diarrhoea. His weight had been on the 25th centile until the age of 9 months, but since then had gradually fallen on to the 3rd centile. His height had always been on the 25th centile. Head circumference, 47 cm (50th centile). Milestones were normal and immunizations given in full.

His father was unemployed and the family had lived with paternal grandparents in council accommodation until recently when they had been asked to leave. Since then they had lived in a squat with very poor facilities.

On examination he was an active, thin but very happy child. No abnormality could be found except for gross nystagmus present in all directions. He was seen by an ophthalmologist who thought the fundi looked normal and diagnosed congenital nystagmus of unknown aetiology.

Following admission to hospital he remained a poor feeder. His mother was encouraged to feed him frequently. She had already delivered at 7 months, the baby being in another hospital. Tube feeding was started because of poor weight gain, with a small degree of success. Extra calories were added to a milk-based feed. Since the parents were agitating to go home, the tube was removed and frequent feeds given by the nurses. Despite adequate calorie intake, the weight remained static. On discharge of the premature baby, the parents insisted on having both children at home. Following discharge he started to lose weight again, the parents had not made up feeds as instructed, and were not feeding him on a regular basis. Despite his emaciation he remained an active, happy child.

Investigations

Hb, 12.2 g. 100 ml^{-1}.
WBC: 13.9 × 10^9. ℓ^{-1}, film, normal.
Urea, 3.7 mmol. ℓ^{-1}.
Sodium, 139 mmol. ℓ^{-1}.
Potassium, 4.2 mmol. ℓ^{-1}.
Bicarbonate, 21 mmol. ℓ^{-1}.
pH, 7.42.
Alkaline phosphatase, 418 IU. ℓ^{-1}.
ALT, 8 IU. ℓ^{-1}.
AST, 20 IU. ℓ^{-1}.
Calcium, 2.30 mmol. ℓ^{-1}.
Phosphate, 1.5 mmol. ℓ^{-1}.

Total protein, 60 g. ℓ^{-1}.
Albumin, 34 g. ℓ^{-1}.
Chest X-ray, normal.
Bone age, just over 1 year.
MSU, NAD.
Stool: semi-solid specimen; micros, no ova or parasites seen; cuture, enteropathogenic *E. coli* 026 isolated.
Xylose level, 1 h absorption test, 2.28 mmol. ℓ^{-1}.
Sweat sodium, 15 mmol. ℓ^{-1}.
Sweat chloride, 4 mmol. ℓ^{-1}.
Urinalysis, NAD.

Questions

1. What three further investigations are required?
2. What is the most likely diagnosis?
3. What is the treatment?

Case 61

A 4-year-old boy is brought to Casualty. He arrived in England 4 days previously, having lived in Turkey for the majority of his life. 2 days ago he had developed a mild fever associated with a cough and headache. Central abdominal pain, apparently dull and constant, had been present for 24 hours and his appetite poor.

He had been born by normal delivery but the length of gestation was uncertain. He was breast fed for 6 months and his weight gain was good. At 9 months he developed a chest infection, and at 2 years had severe gastroenteritis following which he had made slow weight gain for some months. Developmental milestones were within normal limits.

The father works in the Turkish Consulate and the mother is a housewife; both are well. There is one 18-month-old female sibling who had gastroenteritis 2 months previously but is now well.

Examination

Mild pallor.
Throat slightly inflamed.
Cervical lymphadenopathy, nodes small and non-tender.
Tympanic membranes — positive light reflexes.

Chest clear.
Pulse 90/minute, regular; blood pressure 90/60 mm Hg.
Heart sounds normal.
Abdomen slightly distended, mild generalized tenderness, basal sounds present.
Liver 1 cm below the costal margin; no spleen palpable.
Minimal meningism.

Initial investigations

Hb, 9.0 g. 100 ml^{-1}.
WBC: 4.0×10^9. ℓ^{-1} — polys, 25%; lymphs, 62%; eosin., 5%; monos, 6%; basophils, 2%.
Platelets, 203×10^9. ℓ^{-1}.
Throat swab, no growth.
CSF: not under pressure; micros, no cells seen; culture, no growth.
Chest X-ray, clear.
Bilirubin, 34 mmol. ℓ^{-1}.
Alkaline phosphatase, 490 IU. ℓ^{-1}.
AST, 25 IU. ℓ^{-1}.
ALT, 20 IU. ℓ^{-1}.
Urinalysis, NAD.

He is admitted for observation but promptly starts vomiting and the temperature continues on an upward trend. On and off he appears disorientated and on the 4th day after admission he has a generalized convulsion lasting approximately 1 minute. On examination immediately afterwards he is a little drowsy and physical signs appear unchanged. Meningism is difficult to assess, but is not obviously present and the fundi are normal.

Further investigations

Hb, 7 g. 100 ml^{-1}.
WBC: 3.2×10^9. ℓ^{-1} — polys, 22%; lymphs, 60%.
Platelets, 250×10^9. ℓ^{-1}.
CSF: traumatic tap; RBC, 18×10^6. ℓ^{-1}; WBC, 18 polys; 30 lymphs; sugar, 3.3 mmol. ℓ^{-1}.
Blood sugar, 4.2 mmol. ℓ^{-1}.
Calcium, 2.1 mmol. ℓ^{-1}.
Urea, 7.5 mmol. ℓ^{-1}.
Sodium, 134 mmol. ℓ^{-1}.
Potassium, 3.2 mmol. ℓ^{-1}.
Occult test on stools, strongly positive.

Questions

1. What is the most likely diagnosis?
2. Give two investigations.
3. What is the treatment of choice?

Case 62

A 3-year-old boy presents to his general practitioner with pain and a slight limp of his left leg. A week earlier he had had 'flu', consisting of a mild fever, coryza and his being generally 'off colour'. Initially he had appeared to improve, but 2 days previously he had become febrile again with headache and irritability. He complained of pain in the left leg and back the next day, but when he started limping his parents became concerned.

The family were living on a gypsy encampment in a caravan. The camp population was very mobile with many stray animals around. Many of the amenities had been smashed so that lavatories and washrooms provided unsatisfactory sanitation. The father worked in the 'car trade' and the mother was unemployed and illiterate. There were six other children ranging from 4 to 18 years. School attendance had been sporadic. General health was good, but both the grandfather who lived with the family and mother had been treated for tuberculosis some 5 years ago. A couple of children on the camp had also had 'flu'. In the past the patient had been born 'at home', bottle fed and had only been seen twice by a doctor for scabies and tonsillitis.

Examination

Miserable but co-operative child.
Height, 98.7 cm (90th centile).
Weight, 15.6 kg (75th centile).
Pyrexial, 38.2 °C (axilla).
Pulse, 110/min; sinus arrhythmia; blood pressure, 100/60 mm Hg.
Heart sounds, normal.
Chest, clear.
Fauces, mildly inflamed.

Tympanic membranes, normal.
Non-tender tonsillar lymphadenopathy.
Abdomen, normal.
Mild nuchal rigidity.
Pupils equal, reacted to light; fundi, normal.
Cranial nerves, normal.
Left foot drop.
Decreased tone, left leg.
Tender right thigh.
Absent left ankle reflex.
No left plantar reponse.
Sensation normal.

Investigations

Hb, 12.6 g. 100 ml^{-1}.
WBC: 8.3×10^9. $^{-1}$ — polys, 42%; lymphs, 55%; eosin., 3%.
Platelets, 204×10^9. ℓ^{-1}.
Chest X-ray, normal.
X-ray, hips and leg, normal.
Urea, 4.1 mmol. ℓ^{-1}.
Electrolytes, normal.
Blood sugar, 4.2 mmol. ℓ^{-1}.
Calcium, 2.1 mmol. ℓ^{-1}.
Throat swab, no growth.

Questions

1. What is the diagnosis?
2. What two investigations would you do?
3. What three important steps would you undertake in management?

Case 63

A 29-year-old primigravida was admitted at approximately 36 weeks' gestation in early labour. She was experiencing uterine contractions every 10 minutes and had been doing so for the 90 minutes prior to admission. On vaginal examination the os cervix was still closed.

She had attended antenatal clinics regularly after booking in at 12 weeks' gestation. She was 1.5 m tall and weighed 42.2 kg at booking. Weight gain had been satisfactory, blood pressure stable and routine haematology and serology normal, throughout the pregnancy.

Two hours after admission she began to vomit. She was apyrexial and no abnormality was found on examination. Microscopy of urine revealed no WBC or micro-organisms and a peripheral blood film did not show a leucocytosis. An intravenous infusion of 5% dextrose was commenced at 250 ml. h^{-1} and she was given 12.5 mg prochlorperazine as an intramuscular injection. The vomiting persisted for a further 3 hours and then ceased. The intravenous infusion of 5% dextrose was continued at 250 ml. h^{-1} for a further 3 hours, then reduced to 150 ml. h^{-1} until delivery 13 hours later despite an infusion of oxytocin.

She was delivered of a normal male infant who required no resuscitation, birth weight 2.12 kg.

Mother and child were transferred to the postnatal ward. At the age of 3 hours the infant had a generalized convulsion lasting 1–2 minutes and he was transferred to a special care baby unit where an immediate Dextrostix registered 45–90 mg. 100 ml^{-1}.

Examination demonstrated no abnormal or dysmorphic features and he was apyrexial.

Investigations

Hb, 17.3 g. 100 ml^{-1}.
WBC, 14.2×10^9. ℓ^{-1}.
Blood sugar, 7.4 mmol. ℓ^{-1}.
pH, 7.37.
P_{O_2}, 10.7 kPa.
P_{CO_2}, 5.6 kPa.
Bicarbonate, 21 mmol. ℓ^{-1}.
Base excess, $-$ 4 mmol. ℓ^{-1}.
Lumbar puncture: RBC, 4×10^6. ℓ^{-1}; lymphs, 2×10^6. ℓ^{-1}, no organisms seen.
Serum was taken for viral titres.
Bacterial swabs taken from ear, throat, nose, rectum and mother's vagina.

The infant continued fitting intermittently. The convulsions were generalized and short lasting, less than 1–2 minutes. Intravenous diazepam 0.5 mg did not control the fitting.

Questions

1. What is the most likely cause of this baby's fits?
2. Give one vital investigation.

Case 64

A 5-month-old male infant is admitted with diarrhoea and vomiting associated with failure to thrive. He was the third child of an Irish family with two healthy female sibs aged 2 and 5. The family lived in a two-bedroomed council flat on social security.

Birth history was normal, birth weight 3.5 kg. He had no neonatal problems and was bottle fed. He was first admitted at the age of 2 months with loose stools and poor weight gain; weight was 4.2 kg. He was given clear fluids and then regraded on to his usual bottle milk. He gradually gained weight in hospital and was discharged after 10 days. At home he failed to gain any more weight and was readmitted 4 weeks later. A low-lactose milk was substituted and he again started to gain weight. Following discharge he was initially well and cereals were introduced. However, he required further admission with vomiting, loose stools and respiratory tract infection at 4 months. He improved with antibiotics. In view of his continuing poor weight he had the following investigations;
Barium meal and follow-through, normal.
Sweat test: sodium, 35 mmol. ℓ^{-1}.
Jejunal biopsy, minimal villous atrophy with mild non-specific inflammatory changes.

Examination

Length, 60.7 cm (< 3rd centile).
Weight, 4.4 kg (< 3rd centile).
Pyrexial, 38.3 °C (axilla).
Mildly dehydrated.
Pulse, 108/min.
Heart sounds, normal.
Chest: crepitations, right-upper zone.
Abdomen: distended, no tenderness, hepatosplenomegaly, wasting of buttocks.

Investigations

Hb, 9 g. 100 ml^{-1}.
WBC: 10.4×10^9. ℓ^{-1} — neutros, 80%; band cells, 10%; lymphs, 6%; monos, 4%.
Sodium, 130 mmol. ℓ^{-1}.
Potassium, 3.4 mmol. ℓ^{-1}.
Bicarbonate, 16 mmol. ℓ^{-1}.
Urea, 9.2 mmol. ℓ^{-1}.
Calcium, 2.0 mmol. ℓ^{-1}.
Liver function tests, normal.
MSU, no growth.
Stool culture, salmonella species.
Blood culture, no growth.
Chest X-ray, consolidation in the right-upper and middle lobes.

Questions

1. What is the most important investigation to carry out at this stage?
2. What two aspects of treatment for this acute episode would you concentrate on at first?
3. What diagnosis would explain his recurrent problems?

Case 65

A 5-month-old male infant was admitted to the paediatric ward with difficulty in breathing. He had begun to cough 2 days previously and started sneezing the day before admission. He was breast fed but was unable to finish his feeds because of dyspnoea. On examination he had signs of an upper respiratory tract infection and was treated effectively with ½% ephedrine nose drops before feeds. It was then noticed that he had yellow-tinged sclerae. His urine contained no bilirubin and his stools were not pale. Examination demonstrated mild icterus, hepatomegaly to 4 cm below the costal margin but no splenomegaly. Weight, 6.6 kg (25th centile).

Investigations

Bilirubin: 140 μmol. ℓ^{-1}, 80 μmol. ℓ^{-1} conjugated.
AST, 110 IU. ℓ^{-1}.

Alkaline phosphatase, 140 IU. ℓ^{-1}.

The obstetric notes were reviewed. He was born at term, after an uneventful pregnancy, birth weight 3.17 kg. He became mildly jaundiced on day 3, serum bilirubin 180 μmol. ℓ^{-1}, conjugated 40 μmol. ℓ^{-1}. He was discharged on day 7 with no further investigation. He had fed well at home and had gained weight, albeit slowly.

Following the initial post-admission investigations subsequent results revealed:
Bilirubin: 170 μmol. ℓ^{-1}, 140 μmol. ℓ^{-1} conjugated.
AST, 150 IU. ℓ^{-1}.
5-Nucleotidase, 30 IU. ℓ^{-1}.
Alkaline phosphatase, 190 IU. ℓ^{-1}.
Treponema pallidum flourescent antibody titre (FAT), negative.
Blood cultures × 3, negative.
Antibody titres to: Rubella, 1:8; CMV, 1:8; toxoplasmosis, 1:8; herpes virus 1:8.
Reducing substances in stool and urine, negative.
Ultrasound demonstrated an enlarged liver with no other delineated lesion.

The liver enlarged further without concomitant splenomegaly, the urine became dark and contained bilirubin, the stools became pale and putty-like.
Liver biopsy: occasional giant cells, proliferation of bile ductules, inflammatory cell infiltrate.

Questions

1. Give two possible diagnoses.

Case 66

A 3-year-old boy is admitted with a 4-day history of general malaise with dark urine. He had been fit and healthy previously. 24 hours prior to admission he had become jaundiced with itching associated with anorexia and nausea. There had been no change of stool colour and no other symptoms of note. In the past there was no history of consequence and all immunizations had been given apart from pertussis. He was on no medication. The mother was Iraqi and the father Egyptian. There was one 5-year-old female sibling who was well, and they had lived in the UK for several years.

Examination

Height, 87.2 cm (3rd centile).
Weight, 12.9 kg (10th centile).
Miserable, afebrile.
Pale, clinically anaemic.
Marked jaundice.
Pulse, 120/min; blood pressure, 80/60 mm Hg.
Heart sounds, normal.
Chest, clear.
Ears and throat, normal.
Generalized lymphadenopathy.
Abdomen: liver 1 cm, palpable, non-tender; spleen, not palpable.
No abnormal neurological signs.

Investigations

Hb, 5.5 g. 100 ml^{-1}.
Film: fragmented RBC +++, bite cells (Heinz bodies).
Reticulocytes, 12%.
WBC, 20.0×10^9. ℓ^{-1}.
Platelets, 203×10^9. ℓ^{-1}.
Urea, 4.0 mmol. ℓ^{-1}.
Sodium, 134 mmol. ℓ^{-1}.
Potassium, 3.8 mmol. ℓ^{-1}.
Total protein, 58 g. ℓ^{-1}.
Australia antigen, negative.

Questions

1. What is the diagnosis?
2. Give three further investigations you would do.
3. What are four of the most common precipitating factors.

Case 67

A 15-month-old child was seen regularly in Outpatients for recurrent chest infections. He had had several chest infections in the first 7 months, all treated sucessfully by his general practitioner. However, after further episodes, he was referred to hospital.

The chest infections were neither seasonal nor preceded by an upper respiratory tract infection. They had become less frequent since he started walking. Each episode resolved rapidly with antibiotic therapy, but from the age of 5 months, he had had a persistent cough and was noted to wheeze occasionally. He fed well on a mixed diet and drank easily from a teacher beaker. His mother noticed that he had coughing episodes sometimes whilst drinking but he did not lose fluid though his nose. He had one or two bowel actions daily, the stools were brown, not offensive and flushed away easily.

He was born at 37 weeks' gestation, birth weight 2.74 kg. He was transferred to the special care baby unit on day 3 because of choking episodes. All investigations, including a chest X-ray, were normal and he was discharged aged 8 days. Thereafter, he still had occasional coughing episodes whilst feeding and developed his first chest infection aged 5 weeks.

He smiled at 10 weeks, sat unsupported at 7 months and walked at 12 months. He was the first-born child of 'elderly' parents. His father, aged 48 years, was a British Rail 'gang' foreman. His mother, aged 40 years, retained her job as ticket collector. They lived in a privately rented, centrally heated one-bedroomed flat; neither parent smoked.

Examination

Apyrexial.
Height, 75 cm (10th centile).
Weight, 9.5 kg (10th centile).
Pulse, 96/min; sinus arrhythmia.
Heart sounds, normal.
Trachea, central.
Bilateral scattered crepitations and rhonchi in lower zones.
No hepatosplenomegaly.
Cranial nerves, intact.
Coordination, normal for age.
Tone, normal.

Reflexes, normal.
Plantars, downgoing.
Speech: single words used appropriately; no dribbling.

Investigations

Hb, 12.1 g. 100 ml^{-1}.
WBC, 7.3 × 10^9. ℓ^{-1}.
IgG, 7.3 g. ℓ^{-1} (normal range, 3.0–12.0 g. ℓ^{-1}.
IgM, 0.7 g. ℓ^{-1} (normal range, 0.2–1.0 g. ℓ^{-1}).
IgA, 0.3 g. ℓ^{-1} (normal range, 0.2–0.8 g. ℓ^{-1}.
Sweat test, × 2: sodium, 25 mmol. ℓ^{-1}; 21 mmol. ℓ^{-1}.
Stool tryptic activity, detected 1 in 20.
No fat globules or meat fibres seen.
ECG, no abnormalities.
Chest X-ray, patchy shadowing both lower lobes.

Questions

1. Give two possible diagnoses.
2. Give one useful diagnostic investigation.

Case 68

A 27-year-old Latin American woman gave birth, at term, to a female infant weighing 3.752 kg. The pregnancy had been uncomplicated, labour had started spontaneously and the delivery was normal. Mother and infant were well during the immediate postnatal period, so were, therefore, transferred to the ward. The infant was put to the breast immediately and suckled well. At 6 hours of life, the baby had a short apnoeic spell lasting approximately 30 s. She became centrally cyanosed during the episode, but responded to tactile stimuli rapidly. A Dextrostix taken immediately after the episode gave a reading of 0 mmol. ℓ^{-1}. A further breast feed was given, but 15 minutes later the Dextroxtix reading was still 0 mmol. ℓ^{-1}. In view of the earlier symptoms, an intravenous infusion of 10% dextrose was commenced. However, after 15 minutes the Dextrostix reading was between 1 and 2 mmol. ℓ^{-1}.

The mother had lived in England for the past 7 years and was married to an English journalist. There had been no episodes of illness or pyrexia during the pregnancy, nor any known contact with exanthemata carriers.

The first child, born 2 years earlier, had died in the early neonatal period of unknown causes.

Examination

No dysmorphic features.
No petechiae.
No jaundice.
Cardiovascular and respiratory systems, normal.
Marked hepatosplenomegaly.
Not jittery or irritable.

Investigations

Hb, 16.7 g. 100 ml^{-1}.
WBC, 11.3×10^9. ℓ^{-1}.
Blood glucose at time of first Dextrostix, 0.7 mmol. ℓ^{-1}.
pH, 7.29.
P_{O_2}, 11.7 kPa.
P_{CO_2}, 4.8 kPa.
Bicarbonate, 15 mmol. ℓ^{-1}.
Base excess, −9 mmol. ℓ^{-1}.
Lumbar puncture: 12×10^6. ℓ^{-1} RBCs; 0×10^6. ℓ^{-1} WBCs; no organisms seen.
Bilirubin, 4 mmol. ℓ^{-1}.

Questions

1. Give two further helpful investigations.
2. Give a possible diagnosis.

Case 69

A 7-month-old boy is sent for admission by his general practitioner. For the past 3 weeks he has had intermittent diarrhoea and vomiting with a mild pyrexia. He has been treated with clear fluids each time the diarrhoea and vomiting restarted. The fluids were readily taken and the situation improved, but only for a few days when the problems returned. There had been no cough or other respiratory problem.

He was born at term weighing 3.2 kg. He was breast fed and initial weight gain was thought to be satisfactory at the local baby clinic. Since 3 months of age he has had several episodes of pyrexia for which no definite cause had been found. He has been treated with antibiotics on a couple of occasions, with a slow response. He was noted to be frequently miserable, constipated, have a poor appetite, and gain weight very slowly, although still only breast fed. He has had his first triple immunization only, having been ill at other times.

The family are Caucasian and both parents are well. The father is a civil servant and the mother a housewife. There are two daughters, both alive and well.

Examination

Length, 65.1 cm (3rd centile).
Weight, 5.1 kg (< 3rd centile).
Irritable.
Dehydrated with dry mouth and loss of skin turgor.
Mild pyrexia, 38 °C (rectal).
Pulse, 112/min; blood pressure, 65/30 mm Hg.
Heart sounds, normal.
Chest, clear.
Fauces, tympanic membranes no inflamed.
No lymphadenopathy.
Abdomen, normal.
No neurological abnormalities.

Investigations

Hb, 12.6 g. 100 ml^{-1}.
WBC: 11.4×10^9. ℓ^{-1} — polys, 46%; lymphs, 51%; monos, 2%; eosins., 1%.
Sodium, 167 mmol. ℓ^{-1}.
Potassium, 4.8 mmol. ℓ^{-1}.
Bicarbonate, 27 mmol. ℓ^{-1}.
Urea, 7.9 mmol. ℓ^{-1}.
Calcium, 2.4 mmol. ℓ^{-1}.
Plasma osmolarity, 313 mosmol. ℓ^{-1}.

Urine: micros, 3 WBC/mm^3; culture, no growth; ward tests, NAD.
Blood culture, no growth.
CSF: micros; no cells; culture, no growth; protein, 0.45 g. ℓ^{-1}; sugar, 3.1 mmol. ℓ^{-1}.

Questions

1. What is the most likely diagnosis?
2. What two additional pieces of information do you need to confirm your diagnosis?
3. What is the treatment?

Case 70

A 10-year-old boy is admitted with a 5-day history of sore throat, cough, frontal headache and posterior neck pain. He had been seen by his family doctor earlier in the week when a diagnosis of upper respiratory infection was made and co-trimoxazole prescribed. On the day before admission he was seen in Casualty in view of his lack of improvement, and changed onto erythromycin. Over the next 24 hours he had become progressively distressed with difficulty in breathing and with neck pain.

In the past he had had tonsilitis at the age of 5 years but no other major problems. His mother, father and 5-year-old sister had all been well and there was no known infectious contact. They lived in a three-bedroomed council house.

Examination

Height, 143.7 cm (90th centile).
Weight, 31.3 kg (50th centile).
Pyrexial, 38.5 °C (oral).
Distressed, unable to lie down comfortably.
Pulse, 100/min, regular, with marked volume diminution during inspiration.
Heart sounds, normal; no added sounds.
Respiratory rate, 40/min.

Breath sounds, normal; no added sounds.
No other positive signs on examination.

He was observed overnight but the following morning there was no improvement and he was still complaining bitterly of neck pain. On examination he had shallow rapid breathing and on auscultation bronchial breathing could be heard in a small area of the lower anterolateral chest on the right. There was also a rough scratching sound in time with the heart beat heard at the lower left sternal border.

Investigations

Hb, 10.8 g. 100 ml^{-1}.
WBC: 11.8×10^9. ℓ^{-1} — polys, 84%; lymphs, 13%; monos, 1%.
Platelets, 468×10^9. ℓ^{-1}.

Questions

1. What is the diagnosis?
2. What are the three most likely aetiologies?
3. What are the five most important investigations you would undertake immediately?
4. What two lines of treatment would you institute?

Case 71

An 11-year-old West Indian boy was admitted unconscious to the Casualty department. He had been the victim of a school-fight in which four or five older boys had attacked him. He had been beaten to the ground and then kicked repeatedly. By the time the fight was stopped, he was unconscious. On admission to the unit he was breathing spontaneously and there was no airways obstruction. He became semi-conscious within 15 minutes.

He was well known to the Casualty department as he was constantly the victim of school assaults because he was considered abnormal. The school was predominantly white.

He had had one hospital admission for treatment of acute glaucoma.

He was one of seven children; one other brother, also tall, suffered similar school brutality for identical reasons, although five of the seven children attended the school.

Examination

Height, 151 cm (< 90th centile).
Badly bruised face.
Left subconjunctival haemorrhage.
Left ear contused.
Multiple abrasions: right side of face, right hemithorax, right forearm and hand.
Bruising, left hemithorax.
Simple fracture, left forearm.
Pulse, 112/min; sinus arrhytmia; blood pressure, 125/90 mm Hg.
Short mid-systolic murmur.
Pectus excavatum.
Breath sounds, normal.
Tympanic membranes, normal.
Abdomen, soft; no guarding.
Semi-conscious — could respond to questions.
Pupils equal, reactive to light.
Fundi: small area retinal detachment, left lower temporal quadrant.
Reflexes, normal.
Plantars, downgoing.
Joint movement restricted because of pain from assault.

Questions

1. Give two possible diagnoses explaining the chronic abnormalities.
2. Give the urinary abnormality in each.

Case 72

A 24-year-old mother, blood group O, rhesus positive, is delivered of her third son. At birth he is noted to have purpuric spots on the back, in the groin and on the scalp. There are no other abnormal physical signs. He is a full-term, normal delivery following an uneventful pregnancy, weighing 3.64 kg, with an Apgar score of 9 at 1 minute. His two male siblings, aged 2 and 4 years, were both thrombocytopenic at birth, but now are well with normal development and are receiving no treatment.

The mother is a housewife and the father a painter and decorator. Both are Caucasian and there is no family history of note.

Initial investigations

Hb, 13.4 g. 100 ml^{-1}.
WBC, 19.9 × 10^9. ℓ^{-1}.
Platelets, 42 × 10^9. ℓ^{-1}.
Film: reduced platelets, normal appearances of RBC and WBC.
Blood group, ORh–ve.
Direct Coombes' test, negative.

The following day, the platelet count is 39 × 10^9 cells. ℓ^{-1}, but by the third day it has dropped to 17 × 10^9 cells. ℓ^{-1} and the bilirubin level is 145 mmol. ℓ^{-1}.

Questions

1. What is the most likely cause of the thrombocytopenia?
2. What investigation would be most helpful to prove this?
3. What two lines of treatment might you consider?

Case 73

A 5½-year-old girl had been treated for enuresis to no avail by her general practitioner using both the 'buzzer' system and imipramine. She was then referred to a child psychiatrist with similar lack of success over 6 months and so was referred to Paediatric Outpatients to exclude organic pathology.

She had never been dry, either by day or night. The mother had attempted toilet training from 18 months onwards and the child could void a large volume of urine voluntarily, but was damp 10 minutes after micturition and was persistently damp thereafter. She was unaware of passing urine constantly but had bladder sensation and micturated normally. She was continent of faeces. She had never had a urinary tract infection.

She was considered of average intelligence at school, which she disliked because of constant teasing by the other children.

She had two siblings, one aged 8½ years the other 3 years, both of whom were continent.

The parents had been happily married for 13 years and the family lived in a small but comfortable semi-detached house in a garden suburb.

Examination

Height, 111.7 cm (50th centile).
Weight, 19.1 kg (50th centile).
Pulse, 82/min; sinus arrhythmia; blood pressure, 85/60 mm Hg.
Heart sounds, normal.
Kidneys palpable, not enlarged.
External genitalia, normal.
Rectal examination, normal with good anal tone.
Gait, normal.
No sensory loss.
Co-ordination, good.
Reflexes, normal.
Spine, normal configuration.

Investigations

Hb, 12.3 g. 100 ml^{-1}.
WBC, 5.9×10^9. ℓ^{-1}.
Sodium, 131 mmol. ℓ^{-1}.
Potassium, 4.2 mmol. ℓ^{-1}.
Glucose, 4.8 mmol. ℓ^{-1}.
Calcium, 2.3 mmol. ℓ^{-1}.
Urea, 2.0 mmol. ℓ^{-1}.
MSU culture × 3, negative.

Questions

1. What is the diagnosis?
2. Give one investigation to help confirm your diagnosis.

Case 74

A 12-year-old Indian girl is referred to Outpatients by her general practitioner. She has had a dry cough for 3 weeks, starting with a mild pyrexia, sore throat and headache. After 1 week there was no improvement and she had developed crepitations at the right base of the chest. She was given a week's course of ampicillin, but there was no marked improvement so she was changed to co-trimoxazole. 4 days later she developed a mild macular erythematous rash on the trunk and the co-trimoxazole was stopped. The chest signs remained unchanged, she had become anorexic and lost 1.81 kg in weight.

She had been born in India, but the family had moved to England when she was 3 years old. Her previous health was good apart from gastroenteritis age 4 years. There are four siblings, all still living at home; the youngest is aged 5 years. They enjoy good health. The father has recently had a chest infection treated with antibiotics but is now well, working in an Indian restaurant. The mother had tuberculosis shortly after arrival in the UK and has been off treatment and well for the past 7 years. The patient has been fully immunized.

Examination

Height, 1.44 m (25th centile).
Weight, 27.1 kg (3rd centile).
Temperature, 37.2 °C (oral).
Pulse, 92/min; sinus arrhythmia; blood pressure, 110/65 mm Hg.
Heart sounds, normal.
Respiratory rate, 40/min; no cyanosis.
Percussion, dull right base.
Crepitations, right base.
Fauces, injected.
Tympanic membranes, normal.
Small, mobile non-tender tonsillar lymph nodes.
No other positive signs.

Investigations

Hb, 11.4 g. 100 ml^{-1}.
WBC, 6.4 × 10^9. ℓ^{-1} — neutros, 64%; eosins., 2%; lymphs, 30%; monos, 4%.
Urea, 2.3 mmol. ℓ^{-1}.

Alkaline phosphatase, 205 IU. ℓ^{-1}.
AST, 19 IU. ℓ^{-1}.
ALT, 24 IU. ℓ^{-1}.
Chest X-ray: nodular opacities in right lower zone with small right pleural effusion.
Pleural fluid: clear serous fluid; micros, 2 WBC/mm^3; culture, no growth; insufficient for biochemical investigation.
Sputum: upper respiratory tract commensals only.
Mantoux test, 1 in 1000: negative.
Urinalysis, negative.

Questions

1. Give three further investigations to elucidate the diagnosis.
2. Name one drug for the most effective treatment.

Case 75

A 3½-year-old boy was brought to Casualty by his 14-year-old sister. Both parents had full-time jobs, father was a hospital porter, mother a ward domestic, and during school holidays the younger children were looked after by the eldest daughter. All the children had been playing in the local adventure playground that morning when the 3½-year-old began to breathe abnormally. The sister described it as wheezing. This had worsened over lunch time until the sister had become alarmed and brought him to Casualty.

She did not think that he had had any previous serious illnesses. There was no available obstetric or developmental history. The two other siblings aged 10 years and 5 years were healthy and the family lived in a three-bedroomed terraced council house.

Examination

Pyrexial, 38.6 °C (axilla).
Drooling, flushed, centrally cyanosed.

No rash.
Pulse, 132/min.
No added cardiac sounds.
Inspiratory and expiratory stridor.
Respiratory rate, 50/min.
Suprasternal, sternal and subcostal recession.
Breath sounds, normal.
Restless, but appropriately responsive.

Questions

1. Give two immediate therapeutic measures.
2. Give three important investigations.

Case 76

A 6½-year-old boy was playing football in the playground on a hot summer's day, when he suddenly collapsed and became unconscious. He remained comatose for approximately 10 minutes during which time he was motionless. On arrival at hospital he was conscious and complaining of a headache.

He had been previously well and was an active child, playing vigorously with his older siblings. He had never lost consciousness before and there was no family history of epilepsy or migraine.

The birth had been a normal vaginal delivery with a vertex presentation at term. Birth weight was 3.38 kg and there were no neonatal complications. His development was normal. He sat unsupported at 7 months and walked at 11 months. He had coped well during his short period at school.

He was the third child of three. His father was a statistician and his mother was a professional badminton coach. They lived in a well-appointed, four-bedroomed flat. His mother had become depressed 4 months previously and had been prescribed Motival (Fluphenazine and nortriptyline).

Examination

Height, 118.3 cm (75th centile).
Weight, 18.68 kg (10th centile).
Pale, not clinically anaemic.
Pulse, 110 beats/min; sinus arrhythmia; blood pressure, 90/60 mm Hg.
Apex beat, forceful, 5th interspace.
Heart sounds, soft second sound.
Harsh systolic murmur left sternal edge.
Early diastolic murmur, aortic area.
Peripheral pulses, normal.
No radio-femoral delay.
Respiratory, ENT and abdominal systems: normal.
Neurological: fully conscious answered questions appropriately, no nuchal rigidity.
Tone and power, normal and equal in all limbs.
Cranial nerves: normal, no photophobia.
Reflexes, normal.
Plantars, downgoing.

Investigations

Hb, 12.6 g. 100 ml^{-1}.
WBC, 6.7×10^9. ℓ^{-1}; normal differential.
Blood sugar, 7.3 mmol. ℓ^{-1}.
Sodium, 140 mmol. ℓ^{-1}.
Potassium, 3.9 mmol. ℓ^{-1}.
Calcium, 2.43 mmol. ℓ^{-1}.
Skull X-ray, no fractures.
Chest X-ray, no cardiomegaly; lung fields, normal.
Urine and plasma toxicology screen, negative.
Urinalysis, negative.

Questions

1. Give a further vital investigation.
2. What is the most likely diagnosis?
3. Give two further useful investigations.

Case 77

A 42-year-old primigravida was admitted at term in established labour. On vaginal examination the cervix was 5 cm dilated, but the labour then became prolonged and the infant was born following a difficult forceps delivery. The umbilical cord was around the child's neck and required cutting before delivery. Tracheal intubation with IPPV was required for 5 minutes, after which the infant breathed spontaneously. He was noted to be mildly cyanosed; this was presumed to be traumatic cyanosis following the difficult delivery. Nevertheless, he was admitted to the special care baby unit for observation.

The mother had attended antenatal clinic erratically, had refused all medication and continued to smoke approximatley 15 cigarettes and consume at least a half bottle of wine daily. She had continued working as the editor of a well-known periodical until 38 weeks' gestation. Her husband, aged 34 years, was a reporter for a daily tabloid. They lived in a luxurious penthouse flat.

Examination

Birth weight, 2.18 kg (< 3rd centile).
Traumatic cyanosis.
Pulse, 140/min; blood pressure, 80/30 mm Hg.
Heart sounds, thought to be normal.
Systolic murmur maximal in pulmonary area.
Pulses, bounding.
Respiratory rate, 34/min.
Chest sounds, normal.
Liver, 1 cm, soft.
Neurological system, normal.

A provisional diagnosis of a patent ductus arteriosus was made and an infusion of indomethacin commenced. The infant rapidly became intensely cyanosed. The infusion was stopped and the child was transferred in oxygen to the intensive care baby unit at the nearby teaching hospital.

Examination

Deep central cyanosis.
Pulse, 163/min; blood pressure, 70/30 mm Hg.

Heart sounds: 1st sound, soft; 2nd sound, single.
Midsystolic murmur in pulmonary area.

Investigations

ECG: sinus rhythm; axis, +110 degrees; left ventricular dominance in praecordial leads.
Chest X-ray; no cardiomegaly, oligaemic lung fields.
 The child was commenced on prostaglandin E and rapidly became less cyanosed.

Questions

1. What is the most likely diagnosis?
2. Give two further useful investigative techniques.

2 Answers and Discussions

Case 1

Answers

1. (a) Sickle-cell anaemia.
   (b) Septic arthritis.
   (c) Pauciarticular rheumatoid arthritis.
   (d) Rheumatic fever.
   (e) Ulcerative colitis.
   (f) Henoch–Schönlein purpura.
2. (a) Haemoglobin electrophoresis.
   (b) Aspiration of the joint space.
   (c) Anti-streptolysin 'O' titre.
   (d) Blood cultures.
   (e) Erythrocyte sedimentation rate (ESR).
   (f) C-reactive protein.
   (g) Anti-staphylococcal lysins.

Discussion

This child is West Indian and presents with anaemia and a monoarticular arthritis of a large joint. The first diagnosis should, therefore, be sickle-cell disease. Homozygous sickle-cell disease often presents in the first year of life as fetal haemoglobin concentration decreases; however, there is a spectrum of severity, including haemoglobin C and D disease, so initial presentation at this age is feasible. Haemoglobin electrophoresis is, therefore, indicated.

Sickle-cell disease may produce protean orthopaedic problems. Presentation in the first year of life with dactylitis of hands or feet is pathognomonic. Thereafter any bone may be affected by a sickling crisis with capillary thrombosis and subsequent infarction. Involvement of the femoral head may lead to aseptic necrosis, and large areas of destruction in the long bones may produce subsequent deformity. Other areas of deformity include the skull, with bossing and widening of the medulla caused by marrow extension. Osteomyelitis can be difficult to differentiate as clinical signs are similar and X-ray changes occur late.

Septic arthritis, although now no longer common, is still a potential complication of any bacteraemia. Many organisms have been implicated, but staphylococcal infection is commonly recognized. The effect of septic arthritis is dependent on age. In the first year of life nutrient arteries pass through the metaphysis to the epiphysis, allowing bacterial extension and sepsis. There is rapid destruction of the joint, but X-ray changes occur late. In contrast, X-ray changes may occur within a few days in the older child; also, the epiphysis is protected by a metaphyseal plate. Aspiration of the joint spaces produces a purulent fluid with a high neutrophil count (greater than 50 000 mm^{-3}) with low glucose concentration. Gram's staining should identify an organism. Prolonged antibiotic therapy is indicated.

The classification of juvenile rheumatoid arthritis is still not uniformly accepted; however, one classification is based on the number of joints involved. Pauciarticular arthritis (affecting four joints or less) is the commonest presentation of juvenile rheumatoid arthritis. Type I mainly affects girls between 1 and 5 years. Rheumatoid factor is negative, but approximately 60 per cent of patients carry anti-nuclear factor, which has a close correlation with chronic iridocyclitis. There is no HLA association except in those who present and remain with a pauciarticular arthritis; they tend to carry the tissue type HLA-D/TMo. HLA B27 is associated with the Type II pauciarticular type. This mainly affects older boys and is frequently associated with the later development of sacroiliitis. Orthopaedic problems include periostitis, joint destruction with subsequent limitation of movement, bony erosions and osteoporosis. Treatment is often a combination of anti-inflammatory agents and surgical correction. The progress of the disease may be followed by sequential measurement of the erythrocyte sedimentation rate or C-reactive protein.

Rheumatic fever is a possible, albeit rare, diagnosis despite the absence of a preceding illness. Evidence of recent streptococcal infection would be afforded by a raised anti-streptolysin 'O' titre (ASOT) or other anti-streptococcal antibodies. Diagnosis is largely clinical and depends on a combination of major and minor signs. Major manifestations are carditis, polyarthritis, chorea, erythema marginatum and subcutaneous nodules; minor manifestations include fever, arthralgia, raised ESR or acute-phase proteins, leucocytosis and a prolonged P-R interval. Diagnosis is confirmed if the patient has one sign from both categories plus a supporting third manifestation. The arthritis of rheumatic fever may initially mimic septic arthritis, but then becomes flitting, with other joints being affected every 2–3 days. Treatment is with antibiotics, anti-inflammatory agents and possibly steroids. The length of bed rest is dependent on the severity of the carditis.

Ulcerative colitis or regional enteritis may produce clinically identical arthritis. Usually only a few joints are involved and the arthritis occurs when the enteric disease is active. However, the child is anaemic and ulcerative colitis can present as an arthritis alone with no bowel symptoms. The prognosis for joint function in either disease is excellent.

Further reading

Ansell, B. A. (1980). Polyarthritis. In *Rheumatic Diseases in Childhood*, Ed. by B. A. Ansell, p. 41. (London; Butterworths)
Ansell, B. A. (1980), Rheumatic fever — A changing scene In *Rheumatic Diseases in Childhood*, Ed. by B. A. Ansell, p. 152. (London; Butterworths)
Sickle-cell Anaemia
Burr, H. F. (1977). Haemoglobin II sickle cell anaemia and other haemoglobinopathies. In *Haematology*, Ed. by W. S. Beck, 2nd edn., p. 179. (Cambridge, Ma.; MIT press)
Lambotte, C. (1978). Disorders of the haemopoietic system. In *Diseases of Children in the Subtropics and Tropics*, Ed. by D. B. Jelliffe and J. Paget Stanfield, 2nd edn., p. 588. (London; Edward Arnold).

Case 2

Answers

1. (a) Visual field testing.
   (b) Lateral X-ray of the skull.
   (c) Assessment of hypothalamopituitary axis with clonidine or insulin tolerance test and thyrotrophin releasing hormone/ luteinizing hormone releasing hormone (TRH/LHRH) injection.
   (d) Thyroxine.
   (e) Computer assisted tomography (CT) scan.

(f) Bone age.
(g) Testicular responsiveness to three injections of human chorionic gonadotrophin.

Discussion

This boy presents two major problems — small stature and delayed puberty which are definitely interrelated. The most common problem is constitutional pubertal and growth delay. This normally results when a child, generally a boy, has been growing along the tenth centile and continuation of the pre-pubertal growth rate into the teen years results in a drop to below the third centile. There may be a similar pattern in other members of the family, and quite often the testes will have begun to increase in size even though there are no other secondary sexual characteristics apparent. Neither of these points are true in this case. Chronic illness such as asthma, Crohn's disease and anorexia nervosa are also causes, but again cannot be blamed here. Very occasionally hypopituitarism is the problem.

In boys and girls, 97 per cent show signs of puberty by their 14th birthday. In boys it is reasonable to wait until their 15th birthday, but then delayed puberty should be investigated. Delayed puberty can be due to hypothalamic, pituitary, gonadal and adrenal causes apart from constitutional.

This boy probably has multiple pituitary hormone deficiencies since short stature is a prominent feature. In isolated gonadotrophin deficiency the patients may be of normal stature or even tall for their age. Anterior pituitary deficiencies relate to the following factors:

(1) Congenital — genetic, midline embryonic defects or haemorrhagic infarction at birth.
(2) Acquired — space-occupying lesions, post injury or surgery, post irradiation, temporary failure due to emotional deprivation or hypothyroidism.

A space-occupying lesion is high on the list here in the region of the hypothalamus/pituitary in view of the morning headaches suggestive of raised intracranial pressure and the previously probably normal growth and development. Investigations should be aimed at simple preliminary tests, i.e. visual field tests and lateral X-rays of the skull to view the pituitary fossa, clinoid processes and presence or absence of calcification. Hypothyroidism due to thyroid disease should be ruled out by doing T_3/T_4 estimations.

After this, an assessment of the hypothalamus–pituitary-target organ axis should be conducted, including an insulin tolerance test with TRH/LHRH stimulation and measuring the glucose, cortisols, growth hormone, prolactin, thyrotrophin stimulating hormone (TSH), luteinizing hormone (LH), follicle stimulating hormone (FSH) and thyroxine values regularly.

To complete the assessment bone age should be done. This would be expected to be delayed in both constitutional small stature and growth hormone deficiency and thus would mainly be helpful in prognosticating growth potential. A CT scan would help in identifying the position and size of a space-occupying lesion. Lastly, testicular responsiveness can be tested to three injections of human chorionic gonadotrophin if stimulation is in doubt after the hypothalamus–pituitary–target organ axis test. Chronically understimulated testes may take longer to respond.

Further reading

Brook, C. G. D. (1981). Adolescence: Delayed puberty. *British Journal of Hospital Medicine*, **26**, 573.
Preece, M. A. (1981). *Clinical Paediatric Endocrinology*, p. 294. (Oxford; Blackwell Scientific)
Paediatric Endocrinology
Bailey, J. D. *et al.* (1978). Short stature. *Medicine*, Series 3, **10**, 465.

Case 3

Answers

1. Congenital adrenal hypoplasia.

Discussion

The most striking abnormality in this child is the electrolyte result, with marked hyponatraemia, hyperkalaemia and uraemia. Causes include the 'sick-cell' syndrome, resulting from septicaemia; vomiting with inadequate salt replacement and aldosterone deficiency or unresponsiveness.

The membrane sodium pump is disrupted in the 'sick-cell' syndrome with subsequent passive diffusion across the concentration gradient of sodium and potassium. However, urinary steriod values will be either normal or raised, not decreased. The same argument obtains for vomiting with inadequate salt replacement.

The most likely diagnosis is, therefore, an aldosterone dysfunction. In the salt-losing crisis in pseudohypoaldostenorism, urinary steroid metabolites will be normal. During crises in secondary congenital adrenal hyperplasia, urinary steriod precursor metabolities such as pregnanetriol will be raised, except in enzyme deficiencies early in sythesis when fetuses are either female or incompletely masculinized males. Massive bilateral adrenal haemorrhage may present in the first 48 hours causing immediate cardiovascular collapse; less catastrophic haemorrhages may have little effect, but calcification may be seen in later life.

The most likely diagnosis is, therefore, congenital adrenal hypoplasia. Congenital adrenal hypoplasia is a rare condition. Inheritance is sex-linked or autosomal recessive, but sporadic cases also occur. Presentation occurs either early, within the first 36 hours of life or later, between 3 and 4 weeks. Early symptoms include apnoeic episodes, gasping respiration, convulsions, vomiting with electrolyte imbalance and abdominal distension. Signs in the older group include vomiting, with diarrhoea or constipation, electrolyte disturbances and shock.

Diagnosis is by detecting low urinary levels of 17-hydroxysteriods and 17-oxosteriods and absent aldosterone. Treatment requires life-long steriod replacement.

In infants fed on cows' milk an extremely rare presentation of intolerance mimics this clinical picture.

Further reading

DiGeorge, A. M. (1979). The endocrine system. In *Nelson Textbook of Pediatrics*, Ed. by V. C. Vaughan, R. J. McKay and R. E. Behrman, 11th edn., p. 1662. (Philadelphia; W. B. Saunders)

Hamilton, W. (1972). Disorders of the adrenal cortex. In *Clinical Paediatric Endocrinology*, Ed. by W. Hamilton, p. 135. (London; Butterworths)

Case 4

Answers

1. Perthes' disease.
2. (a) Tuberculous arthritis.
   (b) Transient synovitis of the hip, especially after streptococcal infections.
   (c) Osteoid osteoma.

    (d) Juvenile chronic arthritis.
3. Healing in 2–3 years.

Discussion

Perthes' disease is an ischaemic necrosis of the upper femoral epiphysis which presents with persistent or variable pain in the hip, often associated with some degree of pain in the groin and knee in a previously healthy child. The commonest ages of presentation are between 4 and 9 years and boys are affected four times as commonly as girls. On examination the child is usually limping with physical signs limited to the affected hip with some loss of movement particularly in flexion, abduction and internal rotation. X-ray changes depend on the stage of the disease. Initially there is a destructive phase where sclerosis is the first radiographic change in the affected head representing dead bone. Diffuse rarefaction of the entire femur may occur. As repair occurs and dead tissue is replaced by fibrous tissue, there will be both radiolucent and sclerotic shadows with fragmentation of the femoral head which becomes smaller and flatter. The femoral head will then gradually enlarge as the femoral ossification centre enlarges and the femoral neck widens, following repair of destructive foci in both the head and metaphysis.

A technetium-99 scan will show decreased uptake over the femoral head since it is avascular and the isotope is used to show 'hot spots' with increased blood supply. The surrounding zone of increased uptake represents some revascularization and repair. Haematological examination is usually normal, but in this case worsening of the condition appears to have been started by upper respiratory tract infections, with a slightly raised ESR. There is a condition of recurrent transient synovitis of the hip following mild episodes of streptococcal infections, where the degree of loss of movement in the hip will vary from acute spasm with loss of all movement to mild restriction. There is no muscle wasting. Transient synovitis of unknown aetiology also occurs and occasionally Perthes' disease appears to follow such an episode. Radiologically there is usually no abnormality in transient synovitis although there may be slight widening of the joint space on the affected side.

Tuberculous arthritis usually causes insidious monoarticular arthritis of the knee, hip or wrist. Pain is the usual symptom together with marked swelling of the affected joint and localized muscle wasting. General health may not be good with low-grade pyrexia, weight loss and possibly some other site of infection causing symptoms. Osteoporosis is the earliest X-ray finding and is followed by erosive changes. Thus the picture presented here is not typical either in symptomatology or in findings.

Osteoid osteoma when placed near a joint can present with acute or subacute recurrent loss of movement. It particularly affects the trochanteric area thus hip problems are common. Radiologically it can be difficult to detect, but widespread osteoporosis and local sclerosis are found and thus could be a possibility here, but most unlikely.

Other benign bone cysts can mimic arthritis; malignancies can give a mixed osteolytic and sclerotic picture. However, the history in this case makes malignancy unlikely.

Juvenile chronic arthritis can present in a monoarticular arthritis usually of knee, ankle or wrist. However, the radiological findings are of osteoporosis in the early stages followed by accelerated epiphyseal maturation. There is 'boggy' soft-tissue swelling of the joint sometimes with constitutional upset and occasionally positive anti-nuclear antibodies. These findings do not fit with the case outlined above.

The prognosis in Perthes' disease is usually good, with gradual healing over 2–3 years.

Further reading

Ansell, B. M. (1980). *Rheumatic Disorders of Childhood*, pp. 18–40. (London; Butterworths)
Caffey, J. (1967). The Bones. In *Paediatric X-ray Diagnosis*, 5th Edn, pp. 904–14. (Chicago; Yearbook Medical Publishers)
Clinical Orthopaedics and Related Research, (1980) **150**. Calve, J., 2–35. The Classic. On a particular form of pseudo-coxalgia associated with a characteristic deformity of the upper end of the femur. Wynne-Davies, R. 12–15 . Some etiologic factors in Perthes' disease. Gershwin, D. H., 16–21. Evaluation and prognosis in Legg–Calve–Perthes' disease. Fisher, R. L., *et al.* 23–29. Isotopic bone imaging. H. H., Bohr, 30–35. Development and course.

Case 5

Answers

1. (a) Urea/creatinine.
    (b) Serum and urine osmolality.
    (c) Blood glucose.
    (d) Urine microscopy and culutre.

(e) Urinary calcium.
2. Psychogenic polydipsia.

Discussion

This child presents with polydipsia and polyuria, diffuse abdominal pain, a dying father and failing school standards. This suggests several diagnoses including diabetes mellitus, chronic renal failure, diabetes insipidus and psychogenic polydipsia.

Diabetes mellitus is unlikely because of the absence of glycosuria, but blood glucose concentration must be measured. Childhood diabetes usually presents acutely rather than over a period of months, with a severely dehydrated child with acidotic hyperventilation.

Chronic renal failure causes polyuria with low urine osmolality secondary to tubular damage, with a poor response to antidiuretic hormone (ADH). This may also be induced by hypokalaemia, hypercalcaemia or by renal infections. Both electrolytes mentioined are at normal values and there is no history of episodes of weakness suggestive of periodic hypokalaemia. There is no history of overt renal or urinary tract infections, her blood pressure is normal, she is on the 25th centile for both height and weight and the tubules are capable of responding to ADH. Chronic renal failure is, therefore, unlikely. Diabetes insipidus is either hypothalamic or nephrogenic in origin. Nephrogenic diabetes insipidus is sex-linked recessive and is, therefore, confined to males. However, there are individual cases of affected females and some female heterozygotes may demonstrate impaired concentrating ability. Nephrogenic diabetes insipidus usually presents in infancy, but later onset can occur. Symptoms include dehydration, fever, failure to thrive, vomiting and constipation. Mental retardation may be induced. The lesion appears to end-organ failure rather than the production of an abnormal hormone, or rapid inactivation. Treatment is with thiazide diuretics which are thought to act by inducing sodium depletion with subsequent increased sodium reabsorption in the proximal tubules with antidiuretic effect.

Differentiation between hypothalamic and nephrogenic diabetes insipidus is achieved by administering ADH which produces a concentrated urine in those with a hypothalamic lesion. Also the urine osmolality in hypothalamic diabetes insipidus is generally between 50 and 200 mosmol. ℓ^{-1}, whereas that in nephrogenic is between 80 and 120 mosmol. ℓ^{-1}.

Hypothalamic diabetes insipidus and psychogenic polydipsia are differentiated by the water deprivation test. If the problem is psychogenic, urine osmolality should reach 869–1309 mosmol. ℓ^{-1}; however, if the problem is long-standing, there may be inadequate response to ADH with poor concentrating ability.

The urine may become more concentrated during dehydration in hypothalamic diabetes insipidus, but can only reach a maximum of 285 mosmol. ℓ^{-1} which excludes the diagnosis in this case. An alternative differentiating investigation is to infuse hypertonic sodium chloride. In normal children, a urine of smaller volume and greater osmolality will be passed. Those with hypothalamic diabetes insipidus will show neither change. In this case, with poor concentration it would be reasonable to repeat the water deprivation test.

Hypothalamic diabetes insipidus may be either idiopathic, which is more common, or secondary to local pathology. These disorders include intracranial tumours — such as craniopharyngioma, optic glioma, and histiocytosis X — encephalitis and severe head injury. Rarer causes include toxoplasmosis, leukaemia and cerebral haemorrhage. Investigations will be directed towards differentiating these causes. The inheritance of idiopathic hypothalamic diabetes insipidus is sporadic, autosomal dominant or sex-linked recessive. Treatment is with Pitressin (ADH), either given intramuscularly or as a snuff, or with the synthetic arginine ADH desamino-cys-d-arginine-8-vasopressin (ADH DDAVP).

Psychogenic polydipsia is the most likely diagnosis in this child. She presents with vague diffuse abdominal pain, her adoptive father is dying and her school performance is suffering. She has reduced concentrating ability but is able to produce a urine of greater osmolality than is possible in diabetes insipidus. Psychogenic polydipsia is a symptom of a plethora of emotional disturbances and treatment is either individual or family psychotherapy.

Further reading

Anthony, E. J. (1967). Psychiatric disorders of childhood, psychoneurotic, psychophysiological and personality disorders. In *Comprehensive Textbook of Psychiatry*, Ed. by A. M. Freedman and H. I. Kaplan, p. 1401. (Baltimore; Williams and Wilkins)

Chantler, C. (1979). The kidney. In *Clinical Paediatric Physiology*, Ed. by S. Godfrey and J. D. Baum, p. 377 (Oxford; Blackwell Scientific Publications)

Houston, I. B. (1978). Disorders of the urogenital system. In *Textbook of Paediatrics*, Ed. by J. O. Forfar and G. C. Arneil, 2nd edn., p. 874. (Edinburgh; Churchill Livingstone)

Orloff, J. and Burg, M. B. (1972). Vasopressin-resistant diabetes insipidus. In *The Metabolic Basis of Inherited Disease*, Ed. by J. B. Stanbury, J. B. Wyngaarden and D. S. Fredricksen, 3rd edn., p. 1567. (New York; McGraw Hill)

Robinson, A. G. (1976). DDAVP in the treatment of central diabetes insipidus. *New England Journal of Medicine*, **294**, 507.

Case 6

Answers

1. Reye's syndrome.
2. (a) Blood ammonia.
   (b) WBC.
   (c) Serum salicylates.
   (d) Liver function tests.
   (e) Phenestix test of urine.
   (f) Ferric chloride test of urine.
   (g) Coagulation screen.
   (h) pH.

Discussion

The initial diagnosis in this child would be meningitis. However, the lumbar puncture result is normal. It is possible that the pathological changes had not yet occurred, but other abnormalities such as the hypoglycaemia are not a feature of early meningitis.

Drug intoxication should be considered in any child who presents with altered consciousness. This child was hyperventilating, pyrexial and hypoglycaemic. Salicylate poisoning may induce hyper- or hypoglycaemia, pyrexia via uncoupling of oxidative phosphorylation and hyperventilation via a direct effect on the respiratory centre. This diagnosis should be considered in this case. Definitive proof is provided by serum salicylate levels; rapid suggestion may be gained by using Phenestix in the urine or by the colour change induced by adding ferric chloride to boiled, acidified urine to remove the ketones. Blood pH will depend on the dominant feature: either alkalosis from hyperventilation, or acidosis from a combination of salicylic acid and the blocking of the Krebs cycle with subsequent production of lactic acid. In childhood, acidosis tends to predominate.

Against this diagnosis is hyperreflexia, lack of blood in the vomitus from gastric bleeding and the normal potassium value. Hypokalaemia occurs in salicylate poisoning secondary to alkalosis and to a direct effect on the renal tubule producing potassium loss. Treatment is by emesis if the child is conscious and forced alkaline duiresis, used with extreme caution in childhood, if the serum salicylate levels are dangerously toxic.

The most likely diagnosis in this case is Reye's syndrome. The child had a short history of an upper respiratory tract infection, before vomiting and suddenly becoming comatose. Hypoglycaemia, hyperreflexia and hyperventilation are all features of this syndrome. The definitive investigation is blood ammonia level which is markedly raised. The WBC count may also be suggestive, as there may be leucocytosis of up to 40.0×10^9. ℓ^{-1} with a neutrophilia. The CSF WBC count remains normal.

Jaundice, hepatomegaly and coagulation defects usually occur after a few days and are not presenting features.

Various viruses have been implicated in Reye's syndrome, including influenza A, varicella, echovirus and coxsackie viruses. Aflatoxin has also been implicated, as has paracetomol ingestion.

The brain becomes oedematous without cellular infiltration or demyelination and there is a fatty infiltrate of many tissues, especially the liver, kidneys and myocardium.

Treatment is to reduce the raised intracranial pressure and correct electrolyte disturbances.

Improvement, if there is to be any, is usually apparent within 5–7 days; however, there is an approximately 20 per cent mortality and many survivors have neurological sequelae.

Further reading

Reye, R. D. K. and Morgan, G. (1963). Encephalopathy and fatty degeneration of the viscera; a disease entity in childhood. *Lancet*, **ii**, 749.
Sullivan Bolyai, J. Z., Nelson, D. B. Moreus, D. M. and Shoberger, L. B. (1980). Reye's syndrome in children less than 1 year old: some epidemiologic observations *Pediatrics*, **65**, 627.

Case 7

Answers

1. Lead encephalopathy.
2. (a) Encephalitis, viral.
   (b) Space-occupying lesion.
   (c) Meningitis — particularly tuberculous.
   (d) Drug intoxication.

3. (a) Blood lead level.
   (b) Urinary coproporphyrins.
   (c) Full blood count with film for basophilic stippling.
   (d) X-rays of long bones and abdomen.
   (e) Urine: amino acid chromatography and glucose content.
   (f) Plasma phosphate level.

Discussion

Lead encephalopathy is one of the rare but well-recognized causes of coma and convulsions in a child. It should be included in the differential diagnosis of anaemia, convulsions, mental retardation and severe behavioural disorders. Lead poisoning is more common amongst lower-income groups occurring most frequently in children who live in old houses where there may be lead-containing paint, especially in those children with pica. Young children absorb a higher percentage of lead from their gut than adults and retain more. Studies in young growing animals have shown that diets high in fat and low in calcium, iron and other minerals increase the absorption of lead, and this type of diet is again more prevalent in poor-income families.

This child appears to have undergone a normal delivery with mainly normal milestones. However, sitting unsupported late at 10 months and only babbling and cooing at 8 months suggest some degree of neglect on the parents' part. This is further confirmed by the lack of visits to a baby clinic and the failure to thrive. Persistent pica is particularly associated with inadequate mothering.

The presence and severity of symptoms depend upon the amount of lead ingested and the frequency of pica. The earliest symptoms are hyper-irritability associated with lethargy and anorexia. Sporadic vomiting, abdominal pain and constipation are manifestations of lead colic and are not mentioned in this child. Loss of recently acquired development skills may occur and anaemia is characteristic. Thus behavioural changes can precede insomnia and headaches which frequently herald the onset of lead encephalopathy with convulsions, impairment of consciousness, persistent vomiting and ataxia. Massive cerebral oedema is present, although the classic signs of papilloedema and cracked-pot sound on percussion of the skull may not be present. Peripheral neuropathy is uncommon in the young child but may develop and particularly affects the dorsiflexors of the wrist and feet. Acute lead poisoning may cause a Fanconi type of proximal tubular damage with generalized aminoaciduria, glycosuria and hyperphosphaturia. Hypertension has been reported.

Lead poisoning can also take a more chronic course with recurrent symptomatic episodes which abate spontaneously. In the past up to 45 per cent of mentally retarded children have been reported as having high blood lead levels. Whether this is cause or effect is not known. There is no definite blood lead level when a child becomes symptomatic; it varies considerably from approximately 60 μg 100 ml^{-1} to 250 μg. 100 ml^{-1}. However, in lead encephalopathy the blood level usually exceeds 100 μg. 100 ml^{-1}.

Other tests which should be employed in an emergency to make a diagnosis are:

1. A strongly positive qualitative urinary coproporphyrin test.
2. Microcytic hypochromic anaemia with punctate basophilia or stippled erythroblasts in the bone marrow.
3. Radiopaque flecks in the intestine indicating recent ingestion of lead-containing material. Lines of increased density at the metaphyses of long bones.
4. Urine tests for amino acids and glucose levels, together with hypophosphataemia.

Longer term investigations include increased δ-aminolaevulinic acid in the urine and increased free erythrocyte protoporphyrin (FEP). Lead causes partial inhibition of haem synthesis due to its effect on haem synthetase and δ-aminolaevulinic acid dehydratase. FEP is raised in iron deficiency but values above 500 μg. 100 ml^{-1} packed cells indicate lead toxicity.

Differential diagnosis of a space-occupying lesion and viral encephalitis are the most likely, although the 6 months' history of behavioural changes makes the latter distinctly unlikely. Both generally present with headache and vomiting followed by localizing signs, not present in this case. Diminished reflexes with flexor plantars would be unlikely, upper motor neurone signs are more usual. A pyrexia occurs in lead poisoning either as a result of convulsions or from an intercurrent infection which can spark off the acute encephalopathy. Space-occupying lesions from whatever cause — abscess, subdural or tumour — may result in a temperature. Convulsions are fairly uncommon as a presentation of cerebral tumours in childhood occurring in about 10 per cent of patients. EEG and a CT scan would help in the diagnosis of these two conditions.

In view of the meningism present, meningitis must be considered. This could account for the acute illness, but with signs of raised intracranial pressure, a more chronic illness such as tuberculous meningitis (TBM) should come to mind. This would fit with the failure to thrive, but not with the other acute history. TBM usually has a history of about 2 weeks' drowsiness prior to coma and focal signs. The question of a lumbar puncture is a problem. It is very risky in view of the raised intracranial pressure and certainly the above conditions should be diagnosed by other less invasive techniques. In lead poisoning there is a mild pleocytosis and raised CSF protein value which will help very little in distinguishing it definitely from other conditions.

Lastly, in a comatose child who presents an unusual history (even if it is prolonged) that cannot be accounted for, drug intoxication should never be forgotten. This time it seems unlikely in view of the pyrexia and raised intracranial pressure.

Further reading

Barltrop, D. (1981). Lead poisoning. In *Poisoning, Diagnosis and Treatment*, Ed. by J. A. Vale and J. J. Meredith, pp. 178–85. (London; Update Books)
Chisolm, J. J. and Barltrop, D. (1979). Recognition and management of children with increased lead absorption. *Archives of Disease in Childhood*, **54**, 249–62.
Illingworth, R. S. (1979). *The Normal Child* 7th edn. (Edinburgh; Churchill Livingstone)
Committee on Biologic Effects of Atmospheric Pollutants (1972). Lead, airborne lead in perspective. National Academy of Sciences, 71–177.

Case 8

Answers

1. (a) Abdominal ultrasound.
   (b) Intravenous pyelogram (IVP) with late films, i.e. 6 hours.
   (c) Repeat blood cultures.
   (d) Repeat urine cultures.
   (e) DMSA renal scan.
2. Pyonephrosis/infected right hydronephrosis with ureteral obstruction.
3. (a) Drainage of pyonephrosis and nephrostomy.
   (b) Apropriate antibiotics for infecting organisms that will also cross blood–brain barrier.

Discussion

A mass in the right side of the abdomen in a male baby could arise from kidney, liver, bowel, gallbladder or tumour. Throughout this boy's course in hospital he had no obvious bowel symptoms apart from vomiting which could be accounted for by the urinary tract infection and meningitis; there was no palpable liver or jaundice. Instead he appeared to start with a urine infection, developed meningitis from the resulting septicaemia and then had a swinging temperature suggestive of a collection of pus. Subsequent urine microscopy and culture were negative. When this occurs in a child who appears to have continuing infection an obstructed kidney should be considered. To prove this may be difficult if no ultrasound is available. Intravenous urography should be done, but delayed films at about 6 hours or more are very useful. Sometimes the early films show only one kidney functioning. The same problem will occur in the DMSA renal scan. However, late films may show some contrast taken up on the obstructed side. Ultrasound has the added benefit that if the mass is not kidney, then its origin may be delineated.

Further urine cultures may not be helpful in this situation, but blood cultures may grow the organism. The antibiotics already employed will probably make culture difficult.

An obstructed infected kidney has to be relieved and the pus cultured. Since this child has definitely had partially treated meningitis, it is imperative that antibiotics used are appropriate not only for the urinary tract infection but also cross the blood–brain barrier well. Examples are chloramphenicol, co-trimoxazole or trimethoprim alone and cefuroxime. Further treatment depends on the site of obstruction, its extent and whether it is extrinsic or intrinsic. In this child it was at the pelviuretric junction and required prolonged nephrostomy with a pelvo-ureteroplasty at a later date when the infection was cleared. It is important to try conservative surgery in a younger child and not perform a nephrectomy, since hydronephrosis is often bilateral with presentation at different ages.

Further reading

Edelmann, C. M., Jr. (1978). Editor. Urinary tract infections in infants and children. In *Pediatric Kidney Disease*, p. 1123. (Little, Brown)

Nixon, H. H. (1978). *Surgical Conditions in Paediatrics*. Postgraduate Paediatrics Series, pp. 294–298. (London; Butterworths)

Case 9

Answers

1. Anticonvulsant therapy.
2. Reduce, stop or change anticonvulsant therapy or add the daily requirement of vitamin D.

Discussion

The hypophosphataemia and elevated alkaline phosphatase activity suggest that this child has rickets. Collaborative evidence may be gained from X-rays of an epiphysis, and measurement of 25-hydroxycholecalciferol or parathormone. Aminoaciduria and occasionally glycosuria may be present but may be caused by renal damage in this patient. The two potential causes of rickets in this child are anticonvulsant therapy and renal damage; of these, anticonvulsant therapy is the more likely aetiological agent. Renal damage prevents the phosphaturic effect of parathormone causing hyperphosphataemia. Anticonvulsants, mainly phenobarbitone and phenytoin, cause vitamin-D deficient rickets by hepatic enzyme induction producing an increased breakdown of 1, 25-dihydroxycholecalciferol. The resultant hypocalcaemia induces secondary hyperparathyroidisin which maintains serum calcium at the expense of the skeletal pool. Parathormone has a phosphaturic effect causing increased excretion of phosphate and, therefore, hypophosphataemia.

Ideally, treatment would be to reduce, stop, or alter the anticonvulsant therapy; failing this vitamin D supplements of 400 IU daily should be given.

Further reading

Roll, T. W. and Schleifer, L. S. (1980). Drugs effective in the therapy of the epilepsies. In *The Pharmacological Basis of Therapeutics*, Ed. by A. G. Gilman, L. S. Goodman and A. Gilman, 6th edn., p. 456. (New York; MacMillan)

Sinclair, L. (ed.) (1979). Disorders of calcium and vitamin D metabolism. In *Metabolic Disease in Childhood*, p. 181. (Oxford; Blackwell Scientific Publications)

Case 10

Answers

1. Subacute sclerosing panencephalitis (SSPE).
2. (a) Measles antibody titre.
    CSF measles antibody titre.
    EEG.

Discussion

SSPE usually presents between the ages of 5 and 15 years and is associated with a raised blood and CSF IgG and IgM titres of measles antibody. Clinical presentation may be with organic psychiatric features such as a disordered personality, insidious dementia or psychosis; coarse myoclonus and increasing spasticity following neuronal degeneration and occasionally demyelination is seen on histological examination. EEG changes may be specific. The most distinctive feature is the occurrence of bilateral periodic complexes of high amplitude appearing usually every 5–7 seconds. These complexes coincide with a myoclonic jerk.

In an older child, the number of diseases causing regression are much fewer than in children under 18 months. Possible differential diagnoses in this child include: acute psychosis, minor motor seizures, Wilson's disease, Huntington's chorea or late-onset metachromatic leukodystrophy. Acute psychosis is unlikely in view of the slow onset but certainly may present with the clinical picture of acute encephalopathy. Minor motor status is unlikely to present at the age of 12 years and should not be associated with increasing dementia or behaviour disturbance; mental retardation, however, is a common finding. Both Wilson's disease and Huntington's chorea may present with dementia followed by extrapyramidal signs and choreiform movement in this age group. Younger children with Wilson's disease generally present with hepatic problems. Metachromatic leukodystrophy would be extremely unusual at the age of 12 years; presentation occurs around the age of 1 year with regression, ataxia and increasing spasticity. However, there is an adult form.

There are some very rare inborn errors of metabolism which should be considered when all the above have been excluded. These are:

1. Lafora body disease, a degenerative disease starting with epilepsy, then myoclonus and finally extrapyramidal signs, dementia and bulbar palsy.
2. Hallervorden–Spatz disease, in which pigmented material is deposited in the substantia nigra resulting in athetosis, rigidity and dementia.

Further reading

Bellman, M. H. and Dick, G. (1978). Sub-acute sclerosing panencephalitis. *Postgraduate Medical Journal*, **54**, 587–90.
British Medical Journal, (1979). Subacute sclerosing panencephalitis. *British Medical Journal*, **ii**, 1096.
Cavanagh, N. (1981). *A Scheme of Paediatric Neurological Investigation*. (Geigy Pharmaceuticals)
O'Donohoe, N. V. (1981). *Epilepsies of Childhood*. Post-graduate Paediatric Series, pp. 44–55. (London; Butterworths)
Rose, F. C. (ed.) (1979). *Paediatric Neurology*, 1st edn., pp. 203–205, 589. (Oxford; Blackwell)

Case 11

Answers

1. (a) Lumbar puncture.
   (b) Repeat blood culture.
   (c) Counter-current immune electrophoresis.
   (d) Skeletal survey.
2. (a) Pneumococcal meningitis.
   (b) Salmonella osteomyelitis.
3. Penicillin G (benzyl penicillin) intravenously in high dose for 10–14 days.

Discussion

Pneumococcal infection is common in conjunction with sickle-cell disease, particularly in the first years of life. The increased risk results from a deficiency of serum opsonins against pneumococci and the state of functional hyposplenism secondary to reduced phagocytic and reticuloendothelital functions. This is followed later by repeated episodes of infarction in the spleen. Any child with sickle-cell disease whose temperature does not settle on what appears to be appropriate treatment for a specific infection, and who appears unwell, should be suspected of having pneumococcal meningitis or septicaemia. Approximately 10 per cent of children with sickle-cell disease develop pneumococcal sepsis or meningitis in the first 5 years of life. Pneumococcal meningitis has been reported as being 5–50 times more common in black children than white, and approximately 30 times more common in children with sickle-cell disease than other black children.

Partially treated meningitis should be considered in the differential diagnosis of any child who remains unwell despite antibiotics, with signs of irritability or lethargy even in the absence of any meningism. Confirmation is obtained on lumbar puncture with an increased WBC count in the CSF, and raised protein, while culture is generally sterile. Counter-current immunoelectrophoresis on CSF, blood and urine with appropriate antiserum for pnemococci, meningococci and haemophilus influenzae may help to identify the organism.

Treatment with penicillin in high dosage intravenously for at least 10 days is the treatment of choice. This is important because of the high mortality rate, approximately 25 per cent in these cases.

A differential diagnosis in such a patient with sickle-cell disease is salmonella osteomyelitis. This is unlikely in this case, first because the temperature appeared to respond to penicillin when given parenterally. Secondly, the patient did not have bone pain which is generally an early sign and may follow a veno-occlusive crisis. Even if the pain is not localized there is usually reluctance to move the limb involved. Sickle-cell crisis with abdominal pain is also a possibility and can be difficult to diagnose in a young child. Again there is usually pain and tenderness on palpation of the abdomen. The WBC count is not usually helpful, since it is usually raised in sickle-cell disease with a neutrophilia, thus infection and crisis cannot be distinguished easily.

Further reading

Fraser, D. W. *et al.* (1973). Risk factors in bacterial meningitis. *Journal of Infectious Diseases*, **127**, 271–277.
Green, S. H. and George, R. H. (1979). Bacterial meningitis. In *Paediatric Neurology*, Ed. by C. Rose, pp. 569–581. (Oxford; Blackwell)

Marshall, E. C. and Banforth, J. S. G. The impact of pneumococcal infections in paediatrics. In *Pneumonia and Pneumococcal Infections*. Royal Society of Medicine International Congress and Symposium Series, No. 27. (London; Royal Society)
Willoughby, M. L. N. (ed.) (1977). Abnormalities of haemoglobin synthesis. In *Paediatric Haematology*, pp. 118–124. (Edinburgh; Churchill Livingstone)

Case 12

Answers

1. Neuroblastoma in the cervical sympathetic chain.
2. (a) Urinary catecholamine metabolites.
   (b) Chest X-ray.
   (c) Marrow aspiration.
   (d) Angiography.
   (e) Alpha-fetoprotein.
   (f) Carcinoembryonic antigen.
   (g) Skeletal survey.

Discussion

The combination of gastroenterological symptoms and Horner's syndrome in a child is highly suggestive of a neuroblastoma. Either a primary lesion in the sympathetic chain or a secondary lesion in close proximity could disrupt the sympathetic outflow, causing Horner's syndrome; the chronic diarrhoea is caused by vasoactive intestinal peptide which is variably excreted by neuroblastomas. Hypokalaemia may be induced by persistent diarrhoea.

Diagnosis is confirmed by detecting increased levels of urinary catecholamine metabolites. Carcinoembryonic antigen and alpha-fetoprotein may be detected, usually in disseminated disease. Once the diagnosis has been established it is important to determine the extent of the disease, by such methods as ultrasound, bone scan, bone marrow aspiration and arteriography, as this will be a factor in determining treatment and prognosis.

Neuroblastoma is a relatively common tumour of young childhood, 40 per cent occurring by 2 years, 90 per cent by 10 years. It arises from neural crest cells, permitting a wide variety of clinical sites which is reflected in the protean clinical features and presentations. There may be anaemia from marrow infiltration, lymphadenopathy, hypertensiion, non-specific pain and symptoms such as pyrexia, malaise and vomiting. Bony metastases may present with bone pain and are particularly common in the skull, especially the orbit, causing raised intracranial pressure and ptosis. Deposits in proximity to the spinal column may cause stridor, urinary symptoms, or spinal cord and root compression if infiltration occurs.

Tumours occurring *in utero* may cause hypertension, headache and sweating in the mother. Many other presentations have been documented.

The prognosis depends on age, site, state and differentiation. Good prognostic factors include early staging and stage IVS, young presentation, primaries above the diaphragm and well-differentiated histology, although there are well-documented reports of poorly differentiated tumours spontaneously converting to ganglioneuromas.

The accepted staging is:

Stage I,   confined to site of origin.
Stage II, extending beyond the original site but not across the midline.
Stage III, extending across the midline.
Stage IV, distant metastases.
Stage IVS, stage I and stage II with involvement of skin, muscle liver or bone marrow only.

Treatment for stages I and II is surgery while in stages III and IV chemotherapy followed by surgery is being tried. Stage IVS often remits spontaneously.

Further reading

Evans, A. G., D'Augis, G. J. and Koop, C. E. (1976). Diagnosis and treatment of neuroblastoma. *Pediatric Clinics of North America*, **23**, 161.
Jones, P. G. and Campbell, P. E. (1976). Tumours of the adrenal gland and retroperitoneum. In *Tumours of Infancy and Childhood*, Ed. by P. G. Jones and P. E. Campbell. p. 538. (Oxford; Blackwell Scientific Publications)
Mott, M. G. (1979). The presentation, management and prognosis of solid tumours of childhood. In *Topics in Paediatrics. I. Haematology and Oncology*, Ed. by P. H. Morris Jones, p. 55. (Bath; Pitman Press)

Case 13

Answers

1. (a) Hypovolaemia.
   (b) Arterial thrombosis.
   (c) Peritonitis.
2. (a) Coagulation screen.
   (b) Doppler of leg pulses.
   (c) Aortogram.
   (d) Creatinine.
   (e) Blood culture.
3. (a) Insert CVP line.
   (b) Intravascular volume replacement followed by rehydration.
   (c) Steroids.
   (d) Anticoagulant.
   (e) Penicillin.

Discussion

Abdominal pain in nephrotic syndrome frequently heralds the onset of one of the major complications: hypovolaemia or peritonitis. Peritonitis was unlikely in view of the prolonged history, lack of temperature when off steroids and lack of increasing abdominal signs. Hypovolaemia, on the other hand, was very likely right from the start. It often presents with abdominal pain and vomiting and these, compounded with postural hypotension and cool peripheries, are almost conclusive. However, it is easy to make a diagnosis of relapsed nephrotic syndrome secondary to infective gastroenteritis and feel that things will sort themselves out; but fluid balance in an already hypovolaemic patient should be very carefully watched. Following her progress further, weight loss after admission in a patient with nephrotic syndrome and heavy proteinuria is unusual. The dehydration is depicted by the rise in Hb and possibly urea, although the lack of creatinine level makes it impossible to say whether renal function is compromised. If a patient is thought to have severe hypovolaemia they should be treated with salt-poor albumin, 1 g. kg^{-1}, and, if necessary, plasma infusion. Following volume replacement, which can be judged on CVP, rehydration should be started according to the biochemistry.

The second problem this child presents with is ischaemia of the lower limbs. Initially she could be thought to have just poor perfusion, but the history is typical of an ischaemic limb, i.e. cool temperature, pain and tenderness, lack of sensation, then lack of movement. A hypercoagulability state has frequently been described in nephrotic syndrome — reports of arterial thromboses, femoral vein thromboses after venepuncture and the endless argument as to whether renal vein thrombosis is cause or effect of nephrotic syndrome. In view of the above history a clotting screen should be carried out, Doppler soundings of the pulses obtained especially after volume replacement, and if there is no improvement then the patient should be anticoagulated and an aortogram carried out. In general if thrombosis has occurred, the relevant arteriogram or venogram should be done.

As far as further treatment is concerned, penicillin can be added as a prophylactic against pneumococcal infection after a blood culture and the relapse should be treated with steroids.

Further reading

Baker, M. R. (1979). Two cases of nephrotic syndrome with reversible coagulation defect. *Postgraduate Medical Journal*, **55**, 648 757–61.
Barnett, H. G., Schoeneman, M., Bernstein, J. and Edelman, C. M. (1979). The nephrotic syndrome. In *Pediatric Kidney Disease*, Ed. by Edelmann, C. M., Jr., vol. II, pp. 678–695. (Boston; Little, Brown)
Egan, T. J. *et al.* (1967). Shock as a complication of nephrotic syndrome. *American Journal of Diseases in Childhood*, **113**, 364.
Kendall, A. G., Lohmann, R. C. and Dossetor, J. B. (1971). Nephrotic syndrome; a hyper-coagulability state. *Archives of Internal Medicine*, **127**, 1021
Vahaskari, V. M. (1981). The nephrotic syndrome in children. *Pediatr. Ann.*, **i**, 42–64.

Case 14

Answers

1. Somogyi effect.
2. (a) 24-hour fractional urine collections.
   (b) Blood sugar profile.
   (c) 12-hour fractional urinary free cortisols.
3. (a) Lower the insulin dose.

(b) Change insulin to one with a different time action, or to a mixture of insulins e.g. Actrapid and Monotard.

Discussion

A child whose diabetic control is good, as shown by low glycosuria and glycolysated Hb, who also has episodes of ketosis and hyperglycosuria is probably manifesting the Somogyi effect. This is a phenomenon where hypoglycaemia is followed rapidly by hyperglycaemia as a result of the body over-reacting to the fall in blood sugar. Some children show little or nothing in the way of clinical signs to hypoglycaemia. Night-time hypoglycaemia can be a worry of many parents of diabetic children, and may be very difficult to prove. It can be easy to raise the insulin dose in the face of proven glycosuria. An escalating insulin dose may result as described here. Any insulin with a fast-acting component may produce the Somogyi effect towards the end of the morning, but this child is on a long-acting insulin and one should be aware that glycosuria and ketosis does not always indicate poor control. Improved control should result if the insulin dose is reduced, but a change to a biphasic insulin or one with a slightly shorter duration of action may be better. A further alternative is to mix two insulins, one short- and one long-acting such as Actrapid and Monotard or Semitard. Changing the diet to give a heavy carbohydrate load at night is not a satisfactory course of action, but suggesting high-fibre foods and unrefined forms of carbohydrate should produce a slower and more uniform absorption of carbohydrate from the gut and hopefully smoother control.

The simplest test to try and demonstrate a Somogyi effect is a 24-hour fractional urine test. Urine is collected in four timed intervals. In this child glycosuria should be low during the day but the overnight specimen from 8 p.m. to 8 a.m. should show much heavier glycosuria. This will only suggest but not prove the diagnosis. Home blood glucose monitoring is being used more frequently and could be very helpful here, but would require night-time samples. Urinary free cortisols are a method of assessing the 'stress' caused by an unrecognized episode of hypoglycaemia. Careful timing of the samples may show unexpectedly high urinary cortisols at night.

Further reading

Craig, O. (1977). *Childhood Diabetes and its Management*, Postgraduate Paediatric Series. (London; Butterworths)

Case 15

Answers

1. (a) Blood film for red cell morphology and differential WBC.
   (b) Vitamin E levels.
   (c) Coomb's test.
   (d) Glucose-6-phosphate dehydrogenase (G6PD) level.
2. Haemolysis secondary to vitamin E deficiency.

Discussion

A premature baby presenting with a sudden 5 g. 100 ml^{-1} drop in Hb and a seemingly high WBC is either infected, bleeding or haemolysing. The catch is to believe the WBC count done on a Coulter counter which, in fact, counts the total number of nucleated cells and thus nucleated RBC are included. The clue is the number of polymorphs which on a cursory glance look low, but in absolute numbers are within normal limits. The high percentage of nucleated RBCs indicates very high turnover, i.e. RBC destruction. In a well baby gaining weight infection is unlikely. Intrauterine infection could cause haemolytic anaemia, but in the face of a normal IgM result becomes less likely.

A blood film for red cell morphology is essential. This should demonstrate spherocytosis, elliptocytes, Heinz bodies or fragmented cells if the cause is haemolysis. The possible causes are vitamin E deficiency, red cell shape abnormalities, unstable Hb such as G6PD deficiency unusual in Jamaicans and females, and autoimmune antibodies which may be identified by a Coomb's test. The latter is extremely unlikely in a premature baby with an immature immune system. Apart from vitamin E deficiency, the other possibilities, including blood group incompatabilities, should have become apparent with marked neonatal jaundice.

Vitamin E is an antioxidant. Since glutathione peroxidase and catalase activity is diminished in the fetal red cell there is lessened antiperoxidant protection for the red cell membrane. Vitamin E deficiency compounds this lack of antioxidant protection. Premature babies of less than 36 weeks' gestation and weighing less than 1500 g at birth are prone to vitamin E deficiency. This may be due to fat malabsorption, low levels of vitamin E at birth which progressively fall, or the amount of polyunsaturated fatty acids (PUFA) in the feeds, although this is standardized in most milk formulae. The haemolytic process resolves itself at about 38 weeks when fat absorption improves. Treatment is aimed at supplementing with vitamin E, usually by mouth, and stopping any oxidant compounds, especially iron which will increase haemolysis.

A marked drop in Hb may indicate bleeding, common in the premature baby, but usually taking place in the first 1–2 weeks. With no obvious bleeding point or sign of bleeding, this possibility becomes less likely.

Further reading

Gross, S. J. et al. (1979). Vitamin E and neonatal haemolysis. *Pediatrics*, Neonatology Supplement, **63**, 995.
Klaus, M. H. and Farranoff, A. A. (1979). Haematologic problems. In *Care of the High-risk Neonate*, Ed. by S. Grass, 2nd edn., pp. 350–358. (Philadelphia; W. B. Saunders)
Oski, F. A. and Barness, L. A. J. (1967). Vitamin E deficiency: A previously unrecognized cause of haemolytic anaemia in the premature infant. *Journal of Pediatrics*, **70**, 211.
Paediatrics (1979). Vitamin E: Where do we stand. *Paediatrics*, **63**, 933.

Case 16

Answers

1. (a) Blood pressure.
   (b) Palpable gonads.
   (c) Pigmentation.
2. (a) Congenital adrenal hyperplasia.
   (b) Salt-losing crisis.
3. (a) Urinary 11 oxygenation index.
   (b) Plasma 17-hydroxyprogesterone.
   (c) 17-hydroxyprogesterone urinary metabolites.

Discussion

This child has ambiguous genitalia; the most important diagnosis to exclude, therefore, is congenital adrenal hyperplasia (CAH) as a number of these infants suffer from salt-losing crisis. Pigmentation of the infant would suggest CAH, via increased melanocyte stimulating hormone (MSH) activity secondary either to release of MSH from the pars intermedia of the pituitary, or cross-reaction with adrenocorticotrophic hormone (ACTH). CAH is recessively inherited; it is, therefore, probable that the sibling died from a salt-losing crisis rather than 'gastroenteritis'. Hypertension in the infant would suggest a 17-hydroxylase deficiency in which salt-losing crises do not occur. The commonest enzyme deficiency causing ambiguous genitalia with salt-losing crisis is 21-hydroxylase deficiency. 3β-hydroxysteroid dehydrogerase deficiency may produce a similar situation, but is far less common. The crisis usually occurs during the first 3 weeks of life, so fluid and electrolyte balance must be carefully monitored in the neonatal period. Diagnosis is made by determining excess precursors prior to 21 hydroxylation, such as plasma 17-hydroxyprogesterone. However, this metabolite is high normally during the first 48 hours. Urinary ketosteroids will be increased; however, pregnanetriol, a metabolite of 17-hydroxyprogesterone, may not be increased as the pathway is immature until approximately 6 months of age. A useful diagnostic aid is the 11 oxygenation index, the ratio of 11 hydroxysteroids to 11 deoxysteroids, which is raised in CAH.

Only a percentage of infants with 21-hydroxylase deficiency suffer salt-losing crisis although the enzyme is part of the mineralocorticoid pathway. The reason is unknown; isoenzymes and second gene loci have been postulated. Individual enzyme deficiencies are elucidated by detailed analysis of precursors and metabolites. Life-long treatment with mineralo- and glucocorticoids is indicated.

Palpable gonads are virtually always testes; ovaries rarely migrate outside the pelvis. If gonads are palpable in an apparent female, CAH is a tenable diagnosis. The enzyme deficiency would be 20, 22-desmolase or 3β-hydroxysteroid dehydrogenase deficiency, both resulting in a salt-losing crisis, or 17, 20-desmolase deficiency, not associated with dehydration.

Once CAH has been excluded the diagnosis requires further investigative procedures. Chromosome analysis affords genetic sex; phenotypic sex is judged on both internal and external genitalia, usually localized by radiography.

In males there may be a defect in androgen production either peripherally or, rarely, secondary to hypopituitarism. End-organ unresponsiveness to testosterone, testicular feminization syndrome, results in normal female genitalia in the presence of normal circulating testosterone values.

Female virilization is commonly secondary to CAH; other causes include maternal drugs or virilizing tumour during pregnancy, or idiopathic virilization.

The sexual and psychological management of these children is determined by the best function afforded by the external genitalia.

Further reading

Driver, M. and Danish, R. K. (1979). Intersex problems: their clinical recognition, evaluation and management. With review of 47 patients. *Surgery Annual*, **11**, 403.
Lippe, B. M. (1979). Ambiguous genitalia and pseudohermaphroditism. *Pediatric Clinics of North America*, **26**, 91.

Case 17

Answers

1. A toxicological screen of blood and urine.

Discussion

This child was admitted four times before her death with bizarre, unexplained neurological signs and symptoms. At each admission the signs resolved rapidly without treatment or neurological sequelae. In these circumstances drug-induced illness must be excluded by a toxicological screen for the more common psychotropic drugs. In this case, it may have saved the child's life. Children are notoriously adept at acquiring 'safe' drugs; helpful and more ingenious siblings may also be a source of danger.

The mother was reported as suffering from post-partum depression. Contact with her general practitioner revealed that she had been referred to a psychiatrist, who had prescribed imipramine.

Under further questioning mother admitted deliberately giving the child imipramine as she had felt unable to cope with both children.

Analysis of the stomach contents and blood post mortem revealed high levels of imipramine and desipramine, the metabolite. Signs that should have alerted the practitioner were hypotension, tachycardia, especially supraventricular tachycardia. ECG changes are non-specific, but there may be flattening or inversion of the T wave, mydriasis and sluggish reflexes. Other features include dry mouth and flushed dry skin, hypothermia, blurred vision and urinary retention. Apnoea occurs only with high toxic blood levels.

Non-accidental poisoning of children is little reported as yet, but will probably increase in incidence with increasing awareness. There are also scattered case reports of Munchausen's syndrome by proxy, possibly a related phenomenon. Often one or other of the parents has a psychiatric history. Various hypotheses, including marital dysharmony, have been postulated for this form of child abuse but none substantiated.

Treatment requires long-term psychiatric care of the family, or in extreme cases removal of the child.

Further reading

Baldessarini, R. J. (1980). Drugs and the treatment of psychiatric Disorders. In *Pharmacological Basis of Therapeutics*, Ed. by A. G. Gilman, L. S. Goodman and A. Gilman, 6th edn., p. 418. (New York; MacMillan)
Meadow, R. (1977). Munchausen syndrome by proxy. The hinterland of child abuse. *Lancet*, **ii**, 343.
Watson, J. B. G., Davies, J. M. and Hunter, J. L. P. (1979). Non-accidental poisoning in childhood. *Archives of Disease in Childhood*, **54**, 142.

Case 18

Answers

1. (a) Postictal state.
   (b) Subarachnoid haemorrhage.
   (c) Fresh-water drowning.
   (d) Drug intoxication/poisoning.
   (e) Subdural haemorrhage.
2. (a) Repeat electrolytes.
   (b) Lumbar puncture.

(c) EEG.
(d) Blood gases.
(e) Drug screen.
(f) CT scan.
(g) Carotid arteriogram.

Discussion

In view of the poor history it is difficult to make any diagnosis with certainty. A serious head injury is unlikely with no skull fracture, as is subdural haematoma since there was no lucid interval. Spontaneous cerebral insult such as a bleeding arteriovenous malformation, arterial embolus or thrombus is a possibility, but no focal CNS signs make this less likely. Subarachnoid haemorrhage should result in neck stiffness and sub-hyaloid haemorrhages in the eye, but there are always exceptions, and this should be excluded by lumbar puncture.

Metabolic problems in a child who has been well right up to the period of unconsciousness would appear to be a remote possibiltiy; the blood glucose value is normal. However, there are abnormalities of the electrolytes. These at first glance could represent fresh-water drowning, but on closer examination this seems unlikely. Survivors who arrive for treatment after an episode of near drowning will manifest only transient electrolyte changes, which will revert to normal without specific fluid and electrolyte therapy. In one study victims of fresh-water aspiration had a mean serum sodium level of 138 mmol. ℓ^{-1} and serum potassium level of 3.9 mmol. ℓ^{-1}. The ranges regardless of sea- or fresh-water aspiration were: sodium, 126–160 mmol. ℓ^{-1}; and potassium, 2.4–6.3 mmol. ℓ^{-1}. Most victims die from other factors, probably anoxia and acidosis. Aspiration of as little as 2.2 ml/kg of water in animals produces profound changes in $P\mathrm{a}O_2$, which can be accounted for by a large intrapulmonary shunt with a ventilation/perfusion inbalance. Fresh water is absorbed from the alveoli but causes alteration of pulmonary surfactant followed by atelectasis. Hypoxia continues into the recovery phase for a period of 72 hours or more. $P_\mathrm{a}CO_2$ may rise initially but rapidly returns to normal when the patient hyperventilates. A metabolic acidosis is also persistent and marked, probably due to tissue hypoxia. Thus blood gases could be a valuable investigation. Hb and haematocrit are usually in normal ranges in near-drowning victims; haemolysis does occur but is seldom of such a degree to necessitate specific therapy. None of the above features are present in the patient described, cyanosis was short lived and the blood film was normal, thus it seems possible that the low sodium level was erroneous either through laboratory error or blood taken through an intravenous line; it should be repeated.

This boy could be in a postictal state. However, there is no convincing history, and the fact that he swam to the side of the pool suggests a short-lived episode which would not generally be followed by a prolonged period of drowsiness. The momentary shaking and cyanosis at the pool side and on admission could be shivering. An EEG is the simplest investigation and should show an 'epileptic' focus, although this may be difficult to differentiate from an abnormal wave pattern secondary to cerebral abnormality or insult. Depending on the result it may be necessary to proceed to CT scan and for carotid angiography.

In fact the diagnosis was self-poisoning and was first suspected from the EEG which showed signs of drug toxicity. On regaining consciousness he admitted to taking his mother's Valium (diazepam) and barbiturate sleeping tablets in the lunch hour. This underlines the necessity of always taking blood and urine for a drug screen when a child presents in unusual circumstances, especially when one family member is depressed or known to be on medication, or if the family relationships are unusual. Poisoning may be deliberate on the part of patient or parent.

Further reading

Modell, J. H., Graves, S. A. and Ketover, A. (1976). Clinical course of 91 consecutive near drowning victims. *Chest*, **70**, 231.

O'Donohoe, M. V. (1979). Major Generalized epilepsy (grand mal). In *Epilepsies of Childhood*, Postgraduate Paediatrics Series, pp. 87–94. (London; Butterworths)

Case 19

Answers

1. (a) Erythema multiforme.
   (b) Stevens–Johnson syndrome.
2. (a) Mycoplasma pneumoniae infection.
   (b) Viral, particularly herpes simplex.
   (c) Bacterial infection.
   (d) Drug sensitivity, particularly sulphonamides and penicillin.

3. (a) Attack subsides over 2–3 weeks, giving full recovery.
    (b) Recurrent attacks may occur.

Discussion

This child presents a classic picture of erythema multiforme, which may be precipitated by a wide variety of factors such as viral infections, especially herpes simplex, mycoplasma, bacterial infections histoplasmosis and almost any drug. There are three main clinical varieties. First, the papular form which is the commonest, involving hands, forearms and feet. The lesions consist of heliotrope papules and plaques of variable diameter up to 2 cm. Central discoloration of these plaques produces the characteristic 'target' lesion. Secondly, the vesicobullous form, the skin lesions having these characteristics and the oral mucosa is involved. Thirdly, the Stevens–Johnson syndrome, which is a very severe form of bullous erythema multiforme in which the eyes, mouth and genitalia may also be involved. Two such mucous membranes should be involved to make this diagnosis. There is also a severe systemic upset with either fever, polyarthritis, diarrhoea or pneumonia. Conjunctivitis and photophobia may be marked.

Although this child does not fit neatly into one of these classic varieties, he probably is nearest to the Stevens–Johnsons form because of the mouth and eye involvement together with the severe systemic upset. Other viral infections may give this combination, such as echovirus, but generally the rash would not be so florid. The aetiology in this child was never found despite there being some features of bacterial infection, i.e. polymorph leucocytosis and low CSF sugar values. He probably had a viral infection; there was no history of drug ingestion. Differential diagnosis also includes urticaria, but the lesions were not typical, and dermatitis herpetiformis which is rare in childhood particularly at this age.

Treatment is supportive, and any specific infection is treated appropriately. Offending drugs should be withdrawn, and Stevens–Johnson syndrome treated with systemic corticosteroids. The attack gradually subsides over 2–3 weeks with complete recovery but recurrent episodes may occur.

Further reading

Fry, L. (1973). *Dermatology, an Illustrated Guide*, pp. 117–119. (London; Update Publications)

Juhlin, L. (1980). Stevens–Johnson syndrome. *Medicine*, Series 3, **30**, 1553.

Taaffe, A. G. (1975). The Stevens–Johnson syndrome. *British Journal of Clinical Practice*, **29**, 169–171.

Case 20

Answers

1. (a) Malrotation with intermittent volvulus.
   (b) Duplication cyst of the upper small bowel.
2. Contrast studies of the bowel.

Discussion

There are numerous causes of childhood vomiting, both surgical and medical; however, the abdominal X-ray suggests a surgical cause. The stomach and duodenum were dilated with reabsorption of gas from the distal gut, implying an obstruction in the duodenum or proximal jejunum. This is supported by the vomiting being forceful and bile stained, and also by the metabolic alkalosis.

The recurrent nature of the attacks, without diarrhoea, suggest an intermittent, spontaneously resolving obstruction. Intermittent volvulus secondary to malrotation is, therefore, the most likely diagnosis. Volvulus secondary to a duplication cyst is also a possibiltiy but is far rarer. Volvulus without malrotation is also rare and virtually always presents in the neonatal period. Confirmation can be gained by contrast studies using either air or a water-soluble medium, rather than barium, as infarction with subsequent perforation is a potential complication.

The commonest type of malrotation is limited rotation of the bowel through 180 degrees only, resulting in the superior mesenteric artery and caecum lying anterior to the duodenum. Connections from the caecal visceral peritoneum to the parietal peritoneum, in the right hypochondrium (Ladd's bands) may obstruct the second part of the duodenum, or the gut may rotate around the superior mesenteric artery. Less commonly, the initial 90 degree rotation of the gut occurs, the duodenum lying anterior to the superior mesenteric artery, but, thereafter, variable degrees of rotation or non-rotation occur. Volvulus occurs around the short pedicle of small-bowel mesentery. Rarer causes still are congenital kinks or bends or the bowel spiralling on itself.

Duplication cysts can be either tubular, running some length of the bowel, or small cysts. Obstruction is caused by the gut being stretched over a dilated cyst or by the heavier double bowel rotating around the mesentery. Duplication cysts of the duodenum are rare, but those of the small bowel are more common. If there is communication between the bowel lumen and duplication cyst, bacterial overgrowth may occur with the subsequent blind loop syndrome.

Treatment for these conditions is surgical.

Further reading

Black, J. A. (ed.) (1979). Medical conditions which may mimic an acute abdominal emergency. In *Paediatric Emergencies*. Postgraduate Paediatrics Series, p. 390 (London: Butterworths)
Lister, J. and Rickham, P. P. (1978). Malrotation and volvulus of the intestine. In *Neonatal Surgery*. Ed. by P. P. Rickham, J. Lister and I. M. Irving, 2nd edn., p. 371. (London; Butterworths)
Nixon, H. H. (1978). Intestinal obstruction after the neonatal period. In *Surgical Conditions in Paediatrics*. Ed. by H. H. Nixon, p. 237. Postgraduate Paediatrics series. (London; Butterworths)
Rickham, P. P. and Lister, J. (1978). Duplication of the alimentary tract. In *Neonatal Surgery* Ed. by P. P. Rickham, J. Lister and I. M. Irving, 2nd edn., p. 401. (London; Butterworths)

Case 21

Answers

1. (a) Vascular incident, particularly thrombosis.
   (b) Idiopathic.
   (c) Encephalitis.
2. (a) CT scan.
   (b) Left carotid angiography.
   (c) ECG.
   (d) Skull X-rays.
   (e) Chest X-rays.
   (f) Brain scan.

Discussion

Acute hemiplegia in a young child is not rare and can occur secondary to a surprising variety of pathology. There appear to be very few rules that help point to a specific aetiology. There are both vascular and non-vascular causes: viral and bacterial infections, trauma, immunizations, systemic disease, arteriovenous malformations, cardiac abnormalities, status epilepticus and neoplasms are just some examples.

The classic description was given by Freud of a previously healthy child who suddenly becomes ill from the age of a few months to 3 years. The initial symptoms may be violent — with fever, convulsions and vomiting — or may be slight or insignificant. Infantile hemiplegia is not a disease, but rather a non-specific response of the CNS to multiple and varied conditions. In a significant number of cases, varying in different series up to approximately a third, no specific aetiology is found; arteritis has been blamed secondary to an upper respiratory tract infection or unrecognized trauma to the internal carotid artery in the paratonsillar area.

Onset may also be intermittent or 'stuttering', as in this case, and is classic of thrombosis, although this is unreliable. This child had spontaneous occlusion of the left middle cerebral artery for no apparent reason. The middle cerebral artery is also the usual site for emboli which may come from the heart secondary to infective endocarditis and cardiac arrhythmias, or from a lesion in the lungs. Hence the necessity for cardiological investigations with chest X-ray and ECG. In this case there is no pointer to any cardiological problems, thus echocardiogram should be unnecessary. Embolism, by contrast, usually produces a rapidly developing clinical picture.

Cerebral haemorrhage can present in varied fashion; children with haematological problems such as leukaemia, thrombocytopenic purpura and sickle-cell disease are particularly at risk. Blood usually leaks into the subarachnoid space, causing neck stiffness. Subarachnoid haemorrhage itself is generally secondary to vascular malformations such as arteriovenous malformations, angiomas and aneurysms. A carotid angiogram is obviously necessary for diagnosis of these abnormalities since they may not show up on a CT scan. Carotid angiography in the acute phase is not dangerous in experienced hands. Hypertension should never be forgotten as a cause of cerebral haemorrhage even in a child.

Encephalitis is only occasionally complicated by hemiplegia but in the early stages may be focal and cause a vasculitis. Herpes simplex is the best documented viral cause of focal encephalitis and should be excluded by CT scan, if available, since it causes necrotic areas particularly in the temporal lobe. Other viruses such as enteroviruses, mumps, measles and influenza have been implicated, as has immunization with pertussis, measles and rubella vaccines. The EEG may be helpful but sometimes is non-specific with discharges on the contralateral side to the brain lesion which could be explained on cerebral oedema/ischaemia. The CSF findings in this case would support a viral encephalitis but are not diagnostic and viral screen is negative.

In cases of hemiplegia it is imperative that conditions requiring specific treatment are diagnosed. These include space-occupying lesions — particularly subdural haematoma, brain abscess and tumours — bacterial meningitis and any underlying pathology such as pulmonary sepsis. Subdural haematoma often results from mild injury, but in about 50 per cent of cases there is no history of trauma and no radiographic evidence of a fracture, thus skull X-rays are not always helpful. Features against it in this child are the fairly sudden onset and lack of signs of raised intracranial pressure. Cerebral abscess is also unlikely in view of the sudden onset, lack of pyrexia and site of origin of infection, and the CSF findings. Cerebral tumours are generally infratentorial in children presenting with signs of raised intracranial pressure and cerebellar involvement. Hemiplegic migraine is not usually a problem in this age group, since it generally does not start before puberty. The absence of headache and family history is also against the diagnosis. Migraine should always be kept in mind in a patient with sudden onset, then resolution of hemiplegia. Problems may arise when the patient is aphasic, thus unable to give a history.

Further reading

Isler, W. (1971). *Acute Hemiplegias and Hemisyndromes in Childhood*. (London; Heineman Publications)
Gold, A. P. and Carter, S. (1976). Acute hemiplegia in infancy and childhood. *Pediatric Clinics of North America*, supplement (Pediatric Neurology), 413.

Case 22

Answers

1. (a) Acute lymphoplastic leukaemia (ALL).
    (b) Aplastic anaemia.

(c) Lymphoma — non-Hodgkin's.
(d) Juvenile chronic arthritis.
2. (a) Bone marrow aspiration/trephine biopsy.
(b) Leukaemic markers — immunological and enzymatic.
(c) Skeletal survey.
(d) Lymph node biopsy.
(e) Viral studies including: screen of pharyngeal washings, urine, stool and blood.
(f) Australia antigen.
(g) Autoantibodies (Rheumatoid factor).
(h) Technetium bone scan.

Discussion

The main diagnoses here are ALL and aplastic anaemia. Both these diseases usually present with symptoms and signs of anaemia, thrombocytopenia or neutropenia, i.e. lethargy, malaise, bleeding and infection. In aplastic anaemia there is no organomegaly as is present in this case, making aplasia unlikely. One of the main differences is that leukaemia can present with bone pain due to leukaemic infiltration. A viral infection preceding the onset of aplastic anaemia may produce limb pains, but these should have disappeared prior to the onset of symptoms from aplasia, which should occur 4–6 weeks later. Skeletal survey may reveal periosteal reaction and lytic lesions which do not necessarily correlate with the sites of bone pain. These do not occur in aplastic anaemia. A ^{99}Tc scan could also be done to demonstrate skeletal 'hot spots', i.e. involvement.

When ALL presents with aplasia, bone marrow aspiration is unlikely to yield enough cells to allow any differentiation from aplastic anaemia to be made. A trephine biopsy is mandatory and hopefully a diagnosis can be made. Blood and marrow should be sent for leukaemic markers which are immunological and have characteristics either of T cells, (forming E rosettes), of B cells (having monoclonal surface immunoglobulin), or they react with an antiserum raised against non-T and non-B ALL, i.e. common ALL. Enzymatic markers are important; for example, terminal transferase is positive in common and T-cell ALL, while raised levels of hexoseaminidase isoenzymes are present in common ALL.

Lymph node biopsy may be helpful, especially if lymphadenopathy is marked. Cervical lymphadenopathy, as noted in this case, is common in the presentation of lymphoma, both Hodgkin's and non-Hodgkin's. Bone marrow involvement does occur, but aplasia is unlikely to be the main presentation. Usual signs are more localized lymphadenopathy, mediastinal masses which can be symptomatic with progressive dyspnoea, or palpable abdominal masses. Bone involvement may occur with resulting pain.

About 50 per cent of cases of aplastic anaemia can be attributed to viral infections, chemicals or drugs. Of particular note is hepatitis B infection, thus the presence of Australia antigen is important. Immunological factors may also be important, therefore autoantibodies are relevant.

ALL mimics juvenile chronic arthritis (Still's disease) if bone and joint pains predominate. Systemic involvement with generalized lymphadenopathy, fever, abdominal pain, splenomegaly, together with the raised ESR is also similar, but in this case there was no rash during the fever which occurs in the majority of patients. Aplasia does not occur as a complication and obviously one should be wary of making a diagnosis of juvenile chronic arthritis in such a case without first ruling out leukaemia.

Further reading

Ansell, B. M. (1976). *Rheumatic Disorders of Childhood*, Ch. 4. (London; Butterworths)
Chessells, J. M. (1979). *Presentation and Progress in Childhood Leukaemia*, p. 27.
McElwain, T. J. (1979). Hodgkin's disease. In *Topics in Paediatrics. I. Haematology and Oncology*, Ed. by P. H. Morris-Jones, p. 84. (London; Pitman)
Chessells, J. M. and Powles, R. (1980). Acute leukaemia. *Medicine*, **29**, Series 3, 1477.
Gordon-Smith, E. (1980). Aplastic anaemia. *Medicine*, Series 3, **28**, 1454.
Paediatric Clinics of North America (1976). Oncology. February.

Case 23

Answers

1. (a) Hypoglycaemia.
   (b) Infection.
   (c) Apnoea of prematurity.
   (d) Intraventricular haemorrhage.
2. (a) Blood glucose/Dextrostix.

(b) Blood culture/bacterial swabs.
   (c) Lumbar puncture.
   (d) Chest X-ray.
   (e) Viral IgM antibodies.
   (f) High vaginal swab from mother.
3. Apnoea of prematurity.
4. (a) Continuous positive airways pressure.
   (b) Xanthine derivatives.

Discussion

This infant was premature and also small for dates, the birth weight being below the 10th centile, probably secondary to his mother's smoking habits. Both these factors result in reduced hepatic glycogen deposition, rendering the infant susceptible to hypoglycaemia which may occur in the first 24 hours of life. This must be excluded by Dextrostix with a confirmatory blood glucose estimation.

Asymptomatic hypoglycaemia has a good prognosis for future neurological development; however, symptomatic hypoglycaemia, implying severe cerebral hypoglycaemia, carries a poor prognosis with up to 60 per cent of infants having neurological sequelae. Treatment of asymptomatic hypoglycaemia is with increased intake of oral glucose; symptomatic hypoglycaemia requires prompt intravenous therapy.

Infection is always a hazard in the neonatal period, especially in the premature, whose immune responses are immature. This infant was born after prolonged rupture of membranes, increasing the possibility of infection. Signs of infection include lethargy, poor feeding, apnoeic episodes and convulsions. The temperature may be unstable and the WBC is not helpful in the first 48 hours, varying in a non-specific way. Therefore, other investigations, such as blood culture, lumbar punctures, bacterial swabs and viral titres must be undertaken. This mother did not attend an antenatal clinic so nothing is known of her viral status.

The infant may have congenital pneumonia from infected liquor or an ascending infection, from the mother's vaginal and perineal flora. A chest X-ray may show patchy shadowing or lobar consolidation as opposed to the diffuse 'ground glass' appearance of respiratory distress syndrome. Recently, group B haemolytic streptococcus has become more prevalent in England. It infects the cervix, the infant becoming infected during parturition. A septicaemia results, often with accompanying meningitis and pneumonia. The signs may mimic respiratory distress syndrome; differentiation is made by X-ray. A high-vaginal swab from the mother may reveal the presence of the streptococcus.

Various investigations have been suggested as useful in the early detection of neonatal sepsis. These include ESR, total white cell count, acute-phase proteins and gastric washings for white cell count in prolonged rupture of membranes. All these investigations have too high a false negative rate to be used definitively. The decision to start antibiotic therapy is often clinical.

Intraventricular haemorrhages have been detected in a high percentage of premature infants. The infants do not always have previous pathology, but predisposing factors include prematurity, hypoxia, hypercapnoea and positive pressure ventilation. The symptoms depend on the extent of the haemorrhage; a small intracerebral bleed may be manifest by poor feeding, irritability and apnoea, whereas a major bleed is often fatal. Diagnosis is by ultrasound or CT. Although this child had recurrent apnoeic attacks the history states that the infant was otherwise well, which is against all but the most minor of intraventricular haemorrhages.

Idopathic respiratory distress syndrome may occur in an infant of 33 weeks' gestation; however, there are usually early signs of respiratory embarrassment within the first 4 hours after birth, such as grunting, subcostal recession and flaring of the alae nasi. It is unusual for recurrent apnoea to be the presenting sign of respiratory distress syndrome.

No abnormalities were detected on initial examination, during investigations or subsequently; the most likely diagnosis is, therefore, apnoea of prematurity. The periods of apnoea are short and not accompanied by bradycardia and acidosis; however, it is a diagnosis of exclusion and other causes should be sought.

The infant should be placed on an apnoea alarm mattress and can be stimulated at each apnoeic episode. Alternatively, the infant may be treated with xanthine derivatives, such as aminophylline or theophylline, or with continuous positive airways pressure.

Further reading

Ancona, R. J. (1980). Maternal factors that enhance the acquisition of group B streptococci by newborn infants. *Journal of Medical Microbiology*, **13**, 273.

Dykes, F. D. (1980). Intraventricular haemorrhage. A prospective evaluation of etiopathogenesis. *Pediatrics*, **66**, 42.

Kattwinkel, J. (1977). Neonatal apnoea: pathogenesis and therapy. *Journal of Pediatrics*, **90**, 342.

McCarthy, P. C., Jekel, J. F. and Dolan, T. F. (1978). Comparison of acute phase reactants in pediatric patients with fever. *Pediatrics*, **62**, 716.
Naeye, R. L. (1979). Neonatal apnoea: underlying disorders. *Pediatrics*, **63**, 8.
Sabel, D. and Hanson, L. A. (1974). The clinical usefulness of 'C' reactive protein determination in bacterial meningitis and septicaemia in infancy. *Acta Paediatrica Scandinavica*, **63**, 381.
Siegel, J. D. (1978). Detection of group B streptococcal antigen in body fluids of neonates. *Journal of Pediatrics*, **93**, 491.
Todd, J. K. (1974). Childhood infections: diagnostic value of the peripheral white blood count and differential cell counts. *American Journal of Diseases of Children*, **127**, 810.

Case 24

Answers

1. Varicella encephalitis.
2. (a) Viral titres, acute and convalescent.
   (b) CSF viral titres.
   (c) CT scan.
   (d) EEG.

Discussion

This young girl presents with progressive lower limb paresis with intact, although altered reflexes, papilloedema, headache and pyrexia, 4 weeks after chickenpox. Investigations revealed a leucocytosis and a moderately raised CSF protein value. The main diagnoses to consider are, therefore, varicella encephalitis, Guillain–Barré syndrome and paralytic polio. Lead toxicity from absorption of lead in surma (eye shadow) should also be considered. The combination of intact deep tendon reflexes with paresis argues against polio and Guillain–Barré syndrome. The usual progress in polio is loss of the abdominal and cremasteric reflexes followed by loss of the deep tendon reflexes, then paresis. Guillain–Barré syndrome presents as paresis with absent deep tendon reflexes. Lead toxicity presenting as neurological deficit is documented in childhood, but is rare. The most likely diagnosis is therefore varicella encephalitis.

The presentation of post-infectious encephalitis is extremely varied. Bizarre neurological signs, behavioural abnormalities or convulsions may occur days to weeks after the initial illness. Less commonly motor or sensory changes in cranial or peripheral nerves occur, there may also be vision, hearing or speech disturbances. Varicella encephalitis commonly presents with cerebellar signs such as nystagums, ataxia and tremor. Inappropriate secretion of ADH may occur secondary to the cerebral insult.

Encephalitis is a clinical diagnosis, but corroborative investigative evidence is helpful. Lymphocytes in the CSF may range from tens to several thousands; protein is either normal or moderately raised, glucose is normal. Gram's stain and culture are negative, but useful data may be gained from counter-current immunoelectrophoresis when considering a bacterial meningitis.

An EEG in the acute stages is abnormal, but lacks specificity. CT scan is diagnostic only in herpes encephalitis, when a discrete lesion, often in a temporal lobe, may be demonstrated; but CT will demonstrate diffuse cerebral swelling in other encephalitides.

The histological changes in varicella encephalitis are confined mainly to the white matter. There is a cellular infiltrate, initiated by neutrophils, but subsequently lymphocytes, monocytes and macrophages predominate, producing patchy demyelination. Cellular change is usually confined to swelling; however, satellitosis, shrinkage and neuronophagia may occur. The venules in the affected area may show swelling of the endothelium and thickening of the adventitia.

Treatment is symptomatic only; antiviral drugs, such as Acyclovir and interferon, have yet to be of proven worth in varicella.

The prognosis in varicella encephalitis is relatively good, with a 10 per cent mortality. However, a variable percentage of the survivors have subsequent neurological deficit.

Further reading

Ford, F. R. (1972). Intoxications, metabolic and endocrine disorders, dietary deficiencies and allergies involving the nervous system. In *Diseases of the Nervous system in Infancy, Childhood and Adolescence*, Ed. by F. R. Ford, p. 575. (Illinois, C. C. Thomas)

Ross, E. M. and Bellman, M. H. (1979). Encephalitis and encephalopathy. In *Paediatric Neurology*, Ed. by F. Clifford-Rose, p. 552. (Oxford; Blackwell Scientific Publications)

Case 25

Answers

1. Approximately in the region of T3/T4 — anterior pressure on cord.
2. Chronic granulomatous disease (CGD).
3. (a) Spinal X-ray.
   (b) Myelogram.
   (c) Nitroblue tetrazolium (NBT) test.
   (d) Candida killing test.
   (e) Visual count of ingested particles for phagocytosis.
   (f) Neutrophil motility tests, e.g. skin window.
   (g) Staphylococcal killing tests.
   (h) Aspergillus precipitins.
   (i) Mantoux test.
   (j) Blood smear — myeloperoxidase stain to look for large lysosomes in the polymorphs.
4. (a) Spinal decompression.
   (b) Amphotericin/anti-fungal agent.
   (c) White cell transfusion.
   (d) Physiotherapy.

Discussion

A 'cold' abscess on the chest wall, chest symptoms and signs, together with paraplegia strongly suggest a diagnosis of tuberculosis. However, aspergillus was grown from the abscess fluid. This could have been a contaminant, but has been shown to be pathogenic in several clinical situations recently, for example: asthma, cystic fibrosis and CGD. The presence of aspergillus precipitins will confirm that it is pathogenic and not a contaminant. This child presents with a history dating back to the age of 5 months of recurrent infections including bronchitis, cervical lymphadenitis and perianal abscess together with failure to thrive and hepatosplenomegaly. This is a classic presentation of CGD which may also cause: osteomyelitis including infection of the small bones of the hands and feet; liver and lung abscesses; and granulomatous lesions of major organs, for example antral obstruction of the stomach causing vomiting and obstructive uropathy.

CGD is a defect in the neutrophil whereby it is unable to kill ingested bacteria. This defect is due to a failure of the neutrophil to activate one or more oxidases to consume oxygen to produce superoxide or hydrogen peroxide following phagocystosis.

Hydrogen peroxide stimulates the hexose monophosphate shunt and halides are produced. The interaction of reactive oxygen molecules, myeloperoxidase and halides within phagocytic vacuoles results in effective killing of catalase-containing bacteria. These are staphylococci and enteric bacteria, particularly *Serratia marcescens*. Fungal infections, especially candida and aspergillus, are also common. CGD is best diagnosed by the (NBT) test, where NBT is added to cells and is normally reduced to a black pigment within the polymorphs. In CGD, reduction of NBT does not occur; no black pigment appears in the polymorphs. This test can also be used to detect carriers. The 1 hour survival of bacteria may also be compared with normal. With normal polymorphs less than 10 per cent bacteria remain viable after 1 hour when equal numbers of bacteria and polymorphs are incubated *in vitro*, while 80 per cent of bacteria survive in patients with CGD. The polymorphs also show poor candida killing when tested *in vitro*.

When considering a child with increased numbers of infections, abnormalities of immunoglobulins, T- and B-cell numbers and function and neutrophil function are the three categories to investigate initially. In this case the first two are excluded by normal laboratory results. Neutrophil function can be further subdivided into various categories: chemotaxis defects, opsonization defects, defective ingestion of particles and defective peroxidative intracellular killing of bacteria.

Numerous causes for poor chemotaxis have been found such as malnutrition, hyperalimentation and hyper-IgE syndrome. The lazy leucocyte syndrome, which is associated with moderate neutropenia but a normal bone marrow, is one of the most well known. These patients usually have purulent infections of the skin, subcutaneous tissue and lymph nodes, not generally of the bones as in this case. It is diagnosed by either a skin window test or chemotaxis. In the skin window test a cover-slip is pressed onto an area of skin which has been grazed; the area should abound with polymorphs. Chemotaxis can be measured across two filters in a Boyden's chamber, using radioactively labelled cells. Occasionally there is a defect in chemotaxis in CGD.

Opsonization defects cause sepsis from a wide variety of bacteria such as pneumococcus, streptococcus, meningococcus and *Haemophilus influenzae*. These are all unusual causes for infection in CGD since they are catalase-negative organisms and produce their own hydrogen peroxide, thus assisting their demise within the neutrophil.

Disorders of ingestion may be assayed by monitoring rates of particle uptake by polymorphs; for example, opsonized paraffin oil particles.

CGD, a sex-linked inherited disease, should be screened for by the NBT test as described above. Candida and staphylococcal killing tests can be done as tests of neutrophil function. The neutrophils should be tested in both the patients and control plasma just to check that defective function is not secondary to a plasma abnormality. Myeloperoxidase deficiency in polymorphs will mimic CGD in that there is impairment of ability to kill catalase-positive bacteria and candida, but the NBT test will be negative and absence of the enzyme may be picked up on a blood smear stained specifically for the enzyme.

Chédiak–Higashi syndrome, an autosomal recessively inherited disease, causes partial oculocutaneous albinism with photophobia and rotatory nystagmus together with frequent pyogenic infections. The bacteria are not killed since degranulation is defective within the polymorph; large lysosomes may be seen on a blood smear. Clinically this child does not have these typical features and most infections are due to peroxide-producing (catalase-negative) bacteria in contrast to CGD.

The neurological lesion described is consistent with anterior wedging of the spinal cord at about T3/T4. This is because the arms have intact power and sensation and are supplied from C5–T1. T2 supplies the axilla and is the first intercostal nerve. Since this patient is unable to sit without support, this suggests gross interference with trunk musculature supplied from T2–L3. Joint-position sense and coarse touch are carried in the posterior columns of the spinal cord and are intact, while temperature and pain fibres travel in the spinothalamic pathways in the anterior and lateral columns and are not mentioned as being present. Further investigation of the extent of the lesion should be obtained with spinal X-rays which showed collapse of the vertebral bodies of T2–4, and a myelogram showing the level of block. With such marked paraplegia immediate action is necessary to try to decompress the lesion. This can be done surgically, but active treatment of the aspergillus is most important. Amphotericin is still the only really active agent against aspergillus despite claims made on behalf of other antifungal agents. Since the polymorphs in CGD have defective fungal killing, infusions of white cells help to clear infection in conjunction with appropriate antimicrobial therapy.

Further reading

Baehner, R. L. (1980). Neutrophil dysfunction associated with states of chronic and recurrent infection. *Pediatric Clinics of North America*, May, 377–401.
Landing, B. H. and Shirkey, H. S. (1957). A syndrome of recurrent infection and infiltration of the viscera by pigmented lipid histiocytes. *Pediatrics*, **20**, 431.
Matthews, W. B. and Miller, H. (1972). *Diseases of the Nervous System*, pp. 6–23. (Oxford; Blackwells)
Perry, R. (1981). Laboratory diagnosis of immune disorders. *Medicine*, Series 4, **5**, 221–5.

Case 26

Answers

1. (a) McCune–Albright's syndrome.
   (b) Neurofibromatosis.
2. (a) Skeletal survey.
   (b) Gonadotrophins.
   (c) LHRH stimulation test.

Discussion

The child presents with isolated vaginal bleeding for which local causes have been excluded. She is of tall stature and has an advanced bone age, so premature menarche and precocious puberty should be considered. 85–90 per cent of females displaying precocious puberty have no underlying pathology and are assumed to be constitutional. However, it is most unusual for vaginal bleeding to be the presenting symptom, whereas sexual precocity secondary to McCune–Albright's syndrome characteristically presents with vaginal bleeding. Café au lait spots and polyostotic fibrous dysplasia are two other commonly associated features of this syndrome. Neurofibromatosis is another possible diagnosis.

Confirmation of McCune–Albright's syndrome would be gained by detecting the fibrotic lesions on X-ray. Both diseases are assumed to act centrally to cause sexual precocity, gonadatrophins will be consistently high and stimulation with LHRH should evoke an adult response.

Fibrous dysplasia of bone is subdivided into three types: monostotic, involving one bone only; polyostotic; and polystotic accompanied by café au lait spots and sexual precocity. (McCune–Albright's syndrome).

Monostotic may affect any bone, but frequently involves femur, tibia, rib or facial bone. The polyostotic variety may be segmental, involving several bones in one limb. In McCune–Albright's syndrome the café au lait spots, which have an irregular outline, may be distributed over the affected limb.

McCune–Albright's syndrome affects more females than males and is caused by spontaneous mutation; no female has produced an affected offspring. Sexual precocity is the normal endocrine feature, but cases of hyperthyroidism and diabetes mellitus have been described. The disease often presents in infancy with fractures, but may become apparent as late as the fourth decade. Multiple fractures may result in deformity correctible only by surgery. Curettage and bone grafting of the lesions may be beneficial, especially in the adult as the lesions tend to stabilize in adult life. Rarely, sarcomatous change supervenes.

Precocious puberty, defined as the appearance of secondary sexual characteristics before 8 years in a female and 10 years in a male, or the menarche before 10 years, can be classified as central when the hypothalamus or pituitary gland is assumed to be affected, or peripheral when caused by hormone-secreting tumours. Miscellaneous causes include hypothyroidism and exogenous hormones.

The majority of males but only 10–15 per cent of females have underlying pathology.

Central causes include cerebral tumours, such as pineal tumours in males, tumours of the hypothalamus and of the floor of the third ventricle and neurofibromatosis, also meningitis, encephalitis, cysts and hydrocephalus. Breast development and pubic hair usually appear before menstruation and both the penis and testes are enlarged. Stature is initially tall and bone age considerably advanced, resulting in eventual small stature. Gonadotrophin levels will be high and the LHRH stimulation test will give an adult response.

Underlying pathology should be sought especially in males and very young females. If the cause is constitutional, puberty can be suppressed with medroxyprogesterone or cyproterone acetate.

Peripheral causes include ovarian, testicular and adrenal tumours and gonadotrophin-secreting tumours. Masses may be palpated abdominally or rectally, but it must be remembered that ovarian cysts can be induced by central causes. Tall stature and advanced bone age tend to be less marked than in central causes and the penis enlarges, but the testes remain infantile. Except in gonadotrophin-secreting tumours, gonadotrophin levels will be less and sex-hormone metabolite levels high; in all tumours an LHRH stimulation test will return a pre-pubertal result. Management is to delineate and remove the tumours.

Further reading

Dewhurst, J. (1980). *Precocious Puberty in Practrical Pediatric and Adolescent Gynecology*, p. 118. (New York; Marcel Dekker)
Green, M. (ed.) (1980). Symptoms related to sexual development. In *Green and Richmond's Pediatric Diagnosis*, Ed. by M. Green, p. 386. (Philadelphia; W. B. Saunders)
Savage, D. C. L. and Swift, P. G. F. (1981). Effect of cyproterone acetate on adrenocortical function in children with precocious puberty. *Archives of Disease in Childhood*, **56**, 218.
Tachdjian, M. O. (1972). Bone tumours and tumorlike conditions in Bone. In *Pediatric Orthopedics*, p. 513. (Philadelphia; W. B. Saunders)
Warkany, J. (ed.) (1971). Skeletal disorders of uncertain etiology. In *Congenital Malformations. Notes and Comments*, p. 878. (Chicago; Year Book Medical Publishers)

Case 27

Answers

1. Haemolytic uraemic syndrome.
2. (a) Convulsions.
   (b) Hypertension.
   (c) Cardiac failure.
   (d) Acute cortical necrosis, renal failure.
   (e) Coma/decerebrate rigidity/hemiparesis.
   (f) Retinal haemorrhages/subdural haematoma.
3. Fibrin deposition and thrombi in small blood vessels. (Microangiopathic haemolytic anaemia.)

Discussion

From the initial history and examination this child could have haemolytic uraemic syndrome (HUS) intussusception, septicaemia,

Henoch–Schönlein (H–S) purpura, haemolytic crisis, typhoid or poisoning. However, when the investigations are reviewed, thrombocytopenia does not usually occur in these conditions unless disseminated intravascular coagulopathy (DIC) has occurred whereas it is the normal finding in HUS. DIC is ruled out by the normal prothrombin and partial thromboplastin times. In HUS, observations suggest that intravascular coagulation occurs in every patient, but as an initial, very transient phenomenon. Since most children are seen a few days after onset, the most frequent findings are high levels of fibrinogen and some coagulation factors, occurring as a rebound phenomena. About 50 per cent of children do have a prolonged prothrombin time related to a decrease of factor II (prothrombin). Further episodes of DIC may occur but this is unusual; the damage is generally done at the onset. Thrombocytopenia persits for 7–15 days and is followed by a progressive increase in the platelet count.

Pathologically fibrin thrombi develop in small blood vessels, particularly capillaries, with the kidney as a particular target. Linear deposits of fibrin are found on the endothelial surface of the glomerular capillaries thrombosing them and causing acute renal failure of varying degrees depending on the percentage of glomeruli affected. In this case renal impairment is reflected in not only the raised urea, which could be accounted for by dehydration, but also the raised creatinine. Going back to the original differential diagnoses, renal impairment is unlikely unless there has been an episode of hypotension, or direct renal damage from toxin, haemoglobulinuria or proliferative glomerulonephritis.

The same thrombotic process occurring in the CNS produces mild manifestations in approximately half the patients, with irritability, tremor, ataxia and drowsiness. In these cases meningitis and encephalitis would be further differential diagnoses. However, in some patients the problems are more severe, with convulsions, coma, focal neurological signs, decerebrate rigidity, transient hemiparesis, nystagmus and respiratory depression. Retinal haemorrhages are seen in a third of patients. Subdural haematomas are unusual.

Anaemia is usually severe from the onset with extreme pallor. This, with the renal impairment and damage, causes the hypervolaemic cardiac failure and hypertension seen in these patients. Anaemia obviously occurs after haemolytic crisis and occasionally in septicaemia, poisoning or typhoid, but would not be expected in H–S purpura or intussusception.

Haematuria and proteinuria always occur in this illness but when found may indicate other renal pathology — such as post-streptococcal nephritis, H–S nephritis and nephritis associated with systemic lupus erythematosus (SLE) — which should also be considered. Massive haematuria is present in only 10 per cent of patients; hyaline, granular and epithelial casts are also found in the urine. These findings should help differentiate HUS from non-renal pathologies.

Further reading

Dolislager, D., *et al.* (1978). The hemolytic– uremic syndrome: spectrum of severity and significance of prodrome. *American Journal of Diseases of Children*, **132**, 55–58.
Fong, J. S. C., *et al.* (1982). Hemolytic–uremic syndrome: current concepts and management. *Pediatric Clinics of North America*, **29**, 835–856.
Gianantonio, C. A. (1978). Hemolytic–uremic syndrome. In *Pediatric Kidney Disease*, Ed. by C. M. Edelman, vol. II, pp. 724–36. (Boston; Little Brown)
Lancet (1978). Haemolytic–uraemic syndrome in childhood. *Lancet* **i**, 26–27.
Sorrenti, L. Y., *et al*, (1978). The hemolytic–uremic syndrome: experience at a center in the Midwest. *American Journal of Diseases of Children*, **132**, 59–62.

Case 28

Answers

1. Tuberculous meningitis (TBM).
2. (a) Lumbar puncture. CSF: cells and cytocentrifuge, culture, Ziehl–Nielsen stain, protein and sugar levels.
   (b) Mantoux test.
   (c) Gastric washings.
   (d) CT scan.
   (e) Skull X-rays.
   (f) EEG.
3. (a) Hydrocephalus.
   (b) Convulsions.
   (c) Hypothalamic disturbances, e.g. inappropriate ADH secretion.
   (d) Spinal cord block.
   (e) Cranial nerve palsies.

4. (a) Space-occupying lesion.
   (b) Drug intoxication.
   (c) Encephalitis.
   (d) Meningeal spread of a systemic disease, e.g. SLE, sarcoid, reticulosis.

Discussion

This child's history could fit with any one of the differential diagnoses in answer 4. The features that make TBM the most likely are: the gradual onset with increasing irritability and drowsiness, change of character, lethargy and mild pyrexia — i.e., stage 1 TBM in which the symptoms are fairly non-specific, but these together with hilar enlargement on the chest X-ray make it the most likely diagnosis. The absence of focal signs and raised intracranial pressure make a space-occupying lesion less likely especially with this length of history. Focal signs such as cranial nerve palsies (particularly oculomotor) and hemiparesis occur in both viral encephalitis and TBM. These are also the features of stage 2 TBM as are persistent headaches, drowsiness, neck stiffness, increasing confusion, tremulousness and involuntary movements.

Such complications can make TBM very difficult to differentiate from space-occupying lesions, such as subdural haematoma and cerebral abscess, and viral encephalitis. An EEG in encephalitis may show characteristic features and sometimes a focal abnormality. A CT scan would be more helpful in differentiating a space-occupying lesion. A temporal lesion may be seen in herpes encephalitis, but in other encephalitides a CT scan is unrewarding. In TBM some degree of ventricular enlargement may be present. Sometimes patients can present with convulsions at the onset; this particularly happens before the age of 2 years.

CSF count in viral encephalitis and cerebral abscess may mimic TBM in the early stages i.e. polymorphonuclear leucocytes, later changing almost entirely to a lymphocytosis. Usually the cell count rises to $400 \times 10^6 . \ell^{-1}$ and the protein concentration to 0.8–4.0 g. ℓ^{-1}, while the glucose level falls, sometimes to zero. Ziehl–Nielsen stain is required to identify tubercle bacilli in the CSF and often they are found only after a prolonged diligent search. There are no pathognomonic changes in the CSF in viral encephalitis.

To diagnose tuberculosis, a Mantoux test should be carried out and will be positive in approximately 80 per cent of cases. Gastric washings in young children may be positive but tubercle bacilli are notoriously difficult to obtain from young children. Chest X-ray is abnormal in about 75 per cent of cases. Skull X-rays are unlikely to show any abnormality.

Complications in TBM occur as a result of infection of the meninges, e.g. arachnoiditis, and arteritis causing ischaemia and infarction of areas of the brain/spinal cord. As a result of exudate the CSF circulation may be blocked at the aqueduct of Sylvius or the outlet foramina from the fourth ventricle, causing non-communicating hydrocephalus, or around the basal arteries, causing communicating hydrocephalus. The hypothalamus may be damaged, and inappropriate ADH secretion is a well-recognized complication. The arachnoiditis may mechanically strangulate any of the cranial nerves passing through it, and at a lower level in the spinal cord cauda equina and spinal roots damage may result in a variety of radiculospinal manifestations. Arteritis may also produce a great number of clinical manifestations depending on which part of the CNS is rendered ischaemic.

There are other rare but possible diagnoses. First, any child who presents with an unusual history for which no cause can be found should be screened for drug ingestion. The child may have eaten some poisons or drugs, but the parents may also be guilty of deliberately poisoning the child (Munchausen's syndrome by proxy). Secondly, there may have been meningeal spread of a systemic disease. A reticulosis or leukaemia is the most likely in a child of this age. Cytocentrifugation of the CSF to look at the cells should aid diagnosis.

Further reading

Illis, L. S. (1977). Encephalitis. *British Journal of Hospital Medicine*, **18**, 412.
Kocen, R. S. (1977). Tuberculous meningitis. *British Journal of Hospital Medicine*, **18**, 436.
Meadow, R. (1982). Munchausen syndrome by proxy. *Archives of Disease in Childhood*, **57**, 92.

Case 29

Answers

1. 1 week.
2. Skeletal survey.

Discussion

Transverse fractures in the long bones are usually caused by a direct blow to the limbs; spiral fractures are the normal result of accidental injury. However, there are reports of transverse fractures of the humeri caused by sudden jerking of the upper limbs during play. It is likely, however, that the accident described by the mother would produce a spiral fracture; non-accidental injury must, therefore, be considered and a skeletal survey performed. Survey of this child revealed two rib fractures with callous formation, indicating a previous injury. On further questioning mother admitted to the child abuse which had occurred since the marital disharmony. Non-accidental injury must be strongly suspected in a case of multiple fractures — certainly if the injuries are of different ages — if the explanation is not consistent with the fracture or in certain types of fracture, notably metaphyseal. A small flake of bone is detached at the insertion of muscle or ligament, the injury being caused by shaking or violent longitudinal forces.

Bone pathology, such as osteogenesis imperfecta or Caffey's disease, should be excluded and many would advocate a coagulation screen even in the absence of bruising. Any external injury should be photographed.

The true incidence of child abuse, either physical or emotional, is unknown. It does occur in all social spheres, but only the minority come to medical attention. Several psychological and social surveys have listed factors that predispose to child abuse. A recent survey listed 62 key characteristics which included aspects of the parents' childhood, their attitudes towards each other, their individual child-rearing practices and many social factors. It concluded that any family with 15 or more key characteristics was at high risk of child abuse. This family displays several adverse aspects: both parents were young, the accommodation was poor, income was erratic and inadequate and there was recent marital disharmony. The effect of early maternal bonding and breast feeding is constantly stressed; premature infants separated from their mothers at birth suffer a higher incidence of child abuse, whereas infants breast fed for more than 6 weeks are rarely abused.

Each child-abuse case is managed individually; courses of action are to follow up the child at home with frequent visits, or to place the child on the 'At Risk' register which ensures regular health-visitor or social-worker contact. In more serious cases a 'place of safety' order may be obtained and ultimately the child may be placed in care.

Further reading

Cameron, J. M. and Rae, L. J. (eds) (1975). The radiological diagnosis. In *Atlas of the Battered Child Syndrome*, p. 25. (London; Churchill Livingstone)

Poznanski, A. K. (ed.) (1976). The skeletal system. General considerations. In *Practical Approaches to Pediatric Radiology*, p. 325. (Chicago; Year Book Medical Publishers)

Sharrard, W. J. W. (ed.) (1971). Fractures and joint injuries, part II. In *Paediatric Orthopaedics and Fractures*, 2nd edn., p. 1065. (Oxford; Blackwell Scientific Publications)

Case 30

Answers

1. Hand–Schüller–Christian disease (histiocytosis X).
2. (a) Skeletal survey.
   (b) Skin biopsy.
   (c) Bone marrow aspiration (only 10 per cent of cases positive at presentation).
   (d) Liver enzymes.
   (e) Bone age.

Discussion

This child presents with two of the three classic features of Hand–Schüller–Christian disease — diabetes insipidus and proptosis — the third, lytic bone lesions, can be demonstrated clinically in the skull and on skeletal survey. He also had a typical skin rash which, although more a feature of Letterer–Siwe disease, may be the presenting feature in Hand–Schüller–Christian disease. Hypothyroidism and renal pathology are unlikely on the investigative results. Growth hormone deficiency may present at this age but does not explain the clinical signs and symptoms.

Histiocytosis X is a rare disease classically subdivided into Letterer–Siwe, Hand–Schüller–Christian diseases and eosinophilic granuloma. Letterer–Siwe disease is usually seen in the infant and often has a poor prognosis, eosinophilic granuloma has a good prognosis and that for Hand–Schüller–Christian disease is variable. The clinical overlap of these subdivisions is so great that distinction between them is often not made. There is controversy over prognostication and three other groups have been suggested as more relevant for prognosis.

Group 1, with good prognosis, contains children aged over 2 years with no organ dysfunction; group 2, with intermediate prognosis, contains children under 2 years with no organ dysfunction; group 3, with bad prognosis, children under 2 years with organ dysfunction. Organ dysfunction has greater prognostic significance than organ infiltration.

Treatment also is controversial for the more disseminated forms and recent evidence has suggested that the use of one agent, for example chlorambucil, is more effective than combined therapy. Radiotherapy is useful in eosinophilic granuloma and for other discrete lesions.

Diabetes insipidus may remit with therapy; if not, vasopressin must be administered to the patient.

Further reading

Komp, D. M., Vietti, T. J., Berry, D. H., Sterling, K. A., Haggard, M. E. and George, S. L. (1977). Combination chemotherapy in histiocytosis X. Medical and Pediatric Oncology, **3**, 267.
Lahey, M. E. (1975). Histiocytosis X — an analysis of prognostic factors. Journal of Pediatrics, **87**, 184.
Osband, M. E., et al. (1981). Histiocytosis X. Demonstration of abnormal immunity, T-cell histamine H_2 — receptor deficiency and successful treatment with thymic extract. New England Journal of Medicine, **304**, 146.
Starting, K. A., et al. (1980). Chlorambucil in histiocytosis X — A Southwest Oncology Group Study. Journal of Pediatrics, **96**, 266.

Case 31

Answers

1. Surgical exploration.

2. (a) Strangulated hernia.
   (b) Strangulated or torted testis.
   (c) Infected lymph node.

Discussion

This child had a hot, tender, irreducible inguinal mass. The most common causes in a male infant are an indirect inguinal hernia, which has incarcerated or strangulated, or strangulation or torsion of the testis. However, this case was complicated by a swinging pyrexia, not a feature of the above two diagnoses, and a urinary tract infection. The ultrasound demonstrated abnormalities of the right kidney and ureter, probably the origin of the urinary tract infection but not the explanation of the inguinal mass. Surgical exploration is, therefore, indicated. At operation the inguinal mass consisted of the undescended testis and a distal abscess arising from the vas deferens. The latter showed signs of chronic inflammation and was juxtaposed to the abnormal ureter. An *Eschericia coli*, identical with that in the urine, was cultured from the abscess.

A congenital inguinal hernia, far commoner in males, is more likely to become incarcerated or strangulated than in an adult; it is, therefore, important to correct the abnormality promptly. The venous return from the affected gut is embarrassed, causing congestion, oedema and eventual necrosis. The pressure increases within the inguinal canal and the blood supply to the testis may become compromised, as is the case also in torsion of the testis. If a diagnosis of strangulated hernia or testis is suspected immediate surgical intervention is indicated as attempts to reduce the mass are unlikely to succeed and will only prolong the period of ischaemia. There is considerable risk of a contralateral inguinal hernia or torsion of the testis if either has already been manifest in the infant and elective surgical intervention is indicated in both instances.

Further reading

McKendrick, T. (1978). Infection in the urinary tract. In *Neonatal Surgery*, Ed. P. P. Rickham, J. Lister and I. M. Irving, 2nd edn., p. 547. (London; Butterworths)

Rickham, P. P. (1978). Incarcerated inguinal hernia. In *Neonatal Surgery*, Ed. by P. P. Rickham, J. Lister and I. M. Irving, 2nd edn., p. 301. (London; Butterworths)

Case 32

Answers

1. (a) Intraventricular haemorrhage.
   (b) Pneumothorax.
2. (a) Transillumination of the hemithoraces with a cold light source.
   (b) Diagnostic tap of the suspected hemithorax.
   (c) Chest X-ray.
   (d) Ultrasound of ventricles.

Discussion

The immediate possibility which should be excluded in this infant is the position and patency of the endotracehal tube; these variables were excluded, but the child did not respond. Inhalation is unlikely as the gastric aspirate was negligible; infection is also unlikely as this generally leads to gradual deterioration and the child was on antibiotics. Pulmonary haemorrhage is a possibility, but no blood was seen during intubation and air entry was noted to be good. The two most likely diagnoses are, therefore, intraventricular haemorrhage and pneumothorax.

If a pneumothorax is suspected, transillumination of the hemithoraces allows immediate diagnosis and treatment. Chest X-ray may well take too long so a diagnostic tap of the suspected side, using such clues as deviation of the trachea, displacement of the apex beat and differential air entry, may be given. The last sign, however, may not be as useful as chests sounds are well transmitted in the neonate.

Intraventricular haemorrhage (IVH) is common in this age group and the incidence is increased by PPV. There are four categories of IVH: (1) a small subependymal haemorrhage, usually with slight or no clinical symptoms; (2) with extension into the ipsilateral ventricle there may be little clinical disturbance; (3) with blood in the contralateral ventricle; and (4) with dilatation of the ventricles. The last two categories usually have marked clinical symptoms and may well be fatal.

The aetiology of the IVH is controversial. There is still debate as to whether the haemorrhage emanates from the capillaries or from the venous side, but there is agreement that the neonatal lack of autoregulation of cerebral blood flow is a major factor.

Invasive diagnostic techniques are no longer justified as immediate diagnosis does not influence treatment and non-invasive techniques such as CT scanning and ultrasound are now reliable. Diagnosis is important for the long-term management of these children, as awareness allows informed decisions as to treatment of complications such as hydrocephalus.

Recent work has suggested that the use of ethamsylate in susceptible infants may reduce the incidence of IVH.

Further reading

Baden, H. S., Heijjar, W., Chua, C. and Summer, D. S. (1979). Non-invasive diagnoses of neonatal asphyxia and intraventricular haemorrhage by Doppler ultrasound. *Journal of Pediatrics*, **95**, 775.

Berstein, H. (1979). Intraventricular haemorrhage and hydrocephalus in premature newborns; a prospective study. *American Journal of Roentgenology (CT section)*, **132**, 631.

Donu, S. M., Rolloff, D. W. and Goldstein, G. W. (1981). Prevention of intraventricular haemorrhage in preterm infants by phenobarbitone. *Lancet*, **ii**, 215.

Lon, H. C., Lassen, N. A. and Friis-Harsen, B. (1979). Impaired autoregulation of cerebral blood flow in the distressed newborn infant. *Journal of Pediatrics*, **94**, 118.

Morgan, M. E. I., Benson, J. W. T. and Cook, R. W. I. (1981) Ethamsylate reduces the incidence of periventricular haemorrhage in very low birth weight infants. *Lancet*, **ii**, 830.

Volpe, J. J. (1979). Cerebral blood flow in the newborn infant. Relation to hypoxic-ischaemic brain injury and periventricular haemorrhage. *Journal of Pediatrics*, **94**, 170.

Case 33

Answers

1. β Thalassaemia major.
2. Rates of α- and β-chain synthesis in erythroblasts of fetal blood sample.
3. (a) Transfusion problem — sensitization to HLA and minor blood group antigens.
   (b) Iron overload.
   (c) Hypersplenism.
   (d) Folate deficiency.

Discussion

The diagnosis is β-thalassaemia major. This condition occurs in children of parents who are heterozygotes for the β-thalassaemia gene. In this disorder adult Hb, which consists of two α chains and two β chains, cannot be synthesized. The disorder is one of the regulation of β-chain synthesis rather than an absence of the β-chain genes, and several types of genetic defects are known to occur which determine how much β chain is synthesized. In β° thalassaemia, which is the most severe, there is no Hb A production, while in β+ and β intermedia there is some Hb A production. The consequences of the failure to synthesize Hb A are: a profound hypochromic microcytic anaemia due to failure of red cell haemoglobinization, increased destruction of defective red cells giving rise to splenomegaly and mild jaundice, and a compensatory increase in erythropoiesis resulting in extension of the red marrow throughout the bony medulla, with bony expansion especially prominent in the facial bones and skull, and circulating erythroblasts. The predominant Hb synthesized in thalassaemia major is Hb F (two γ, two α chains) and Hb A2 (two δ, two α chains). In addition there is an excess of α chains synthesized in the red cell which precipitate within it to produce the appearance of basophilic stippling. The thalassaemia gene has a high incidence in people of Mediterranean and Far Eastern origin, and thalassaemia major should be suspected in any child of such parents presenting with a profound hypochromic anaemia in the first year of life. The differential diagnosis is hypochromic anaemia due to iron deficiency, or other Hb variants such as Hb Lepore, Hb E + thalassaemia, α-thalassaemia minor (Hb H disease) which can easily be distinguished by Hb electrophoresis.

The diagnosis is made on the characteristic blood picture of profound hypochromia with microcytes, poikilocytes and ghost-like red cells (leptocytes), together with features of chronic haemolysis: increased unconjugated bilirubin, circulating nucleated red cells, leucocytosis and occasionally reticulocytosis. The diagnosis is confirmed by Hb electrophoresis. There is a predominance of Hb F, Hb A2 is often marginally raised, and there is a variable amount of Hb A production according to the exact gene defect. This patient has β + thalassaemia since there is some Hb A production. Further investigations, such as estimating the rates of β- and α-chain synthesis in the erythroblasts, are usually only applicable as research procedures but can be done on fetal blood samples to distinguish between homozygote (major) and heterozygotes (thalassaemia minor) states.

The management is regular blood transfusion to keep the Hb in the range of over 10 g. 100 ml^{-1}; this will require transfusions every 3–4 weeks. Patients will rapidly develop problems associated with chronic transfusion treatment — sensitization to HLA antigens requiring the careful selection of blood free of minor antigens by the transfusion centre. Desferrioxamine given with transfusion and administered subcutaneously overnight up to 5 days a week continually should be instituted as soon as transfusion is commenced. Regular measurements of serum ferritin will identify whether iron overload is occuring, and folic acid supplements may be necessary in some patients with excessive erythropoiesis. Occasionally splenomegaly may be a problem requiring splenectomy to reduce haemolysis. Splenectomy should be delayed as long as possible to reduce the risk of post-splenectomy immune defects in children under the age of 6 where pneumococcal and *Haemophilus influenzae* septicaemia can occur. Pneumococcal antigen vaccination before splenectomy may be helpful in reducing this risk.

Further reading

Ohene-Frempong, K. and Schwartz, E. (1980). Clinical features of thalassaemia. *Pediatric Clinics of North America*, May, 403–420.
Propper, R. D. (1980). Haemolytic anaemia: thalassaemia syndromes. *Annals of Pediatrics*, **8**, 300–307.
Seattle Bone Marrow Transplantation Group (1982). Bone marrow transplantation for Beta Thalassaemia major. *Lancet*, **ii**, 227–229.
Todd, D. (1980). Thalassaemias and the haemoglobinopathies *Medicine*, Series 3, **27**, 1406–1412.
Willoughby, M. L. N. (ed.) (1977). Thalassaemia syndromes. In *Paediatirc Haematology*, pp. 129–137. (Edinburgh; Churchill Livingstone)

Case 34

Answers

1. (a) CT scan.
   (b) Blood pressure.
   (c) CSF pressure.
   (d) Skull X-ray.
   (e) Viral titres.

2. Pseudotumour cerebri (benign intracranial hypertension) secondary to otitis media.
3. Reduction of the raised intracranial pressure by:
   (a) Hypertonic solutions.
   (b) Surgical decompression.
   (c) Ventriculoperitoneal shunt.
   (d) Repeated lumbar punctures.
4. (a) Addison's disease.
   (b) Cushing's disease.
   (c) Hypoparathyroidism.
   (d) Hyper-hypothyroidism.
   (e) Tetracyclines.
   (f) Steroids.
   (g) Penicillin.
   (h) Pulmonary encephalopathy.
   (i) Infectious mononucleosis.
   (j) High CSF in protein, e.g. polyneuritis.

Discussion

There are numerous causes of raised intracranial pressure in childhood; however, two aspects of this child's history warrant closer attention. The fall may be relevant. However, he was not knocked out and there was no history of head injury, although neither need be present with intracranial damage. However, the history is too long for either an extradural or acute subdural haemorrhage, both of which should cause signs within 24–36 hours. A skull X-ray should reveal a fracture.

The other aspect is the otitis media suffered 2 weeks previously. Otitis media may cause a variety of intracranial complications including meningitis and cerebral abscess. However, the CSF was normal and he had only mild nuchal rigidity and both the 'tripod' and Kernig's signs were negative; he was also apyrexial. The period between presentation and the initial infection is also somewhat long. A likely diagnosis is, therefore, otitic hydrocephalus or pseudotumour cerebri. The mechanism for raised intracranial pressure is thought to be non-septic thrombosis of the lateral venous sinus.

The blood pressure is useful; however, if it is high it may be the cause or the result of the encephalopathy.

Symptoms are those of raised intracranial pressure. There may be a loss of visual acuity from papilloedema and a particularly ominous sign is amaurosis fugax — repeated, transient, episodes of dimming or loss of vision. Diplopia may occur from an abducens palsy.

The CSF in this condition is normal except for the grossly raised pressure.

The time span from the original coryza is consistent with a viral encephalitis. The CSF may be normal, but this child is apyrexial, has a normal white cell count and no lymphocytosis. A CT scan in encephalitis may reveal cerebral oedema or a localized lesion in herpes encephalitis. In pseudotumour cerebri the scan is either normal or shows small ventricles. It may be prudent, if the diagnosis is in doubt, to perform a cisternal puncture or await the CT scan before attempting a lumbar puncture.

The child has markedly raised intracranial pressure as evidenced by papilloedema and a VIth nerve palsy; urgent treatment is, therefore, required. Cerebral oedema is not a feature of this syndrome; however, hypertonic solutions may reduce the intracranial pressure rapidly. Other approaches include repeated lumbar punctures, surgical decompression or a ventriculoperitoneal shunt. However, as the ventricles are normal or small, positioning the shunt may be difficult. This condition may last several months, but usually resolves spontaneously and has a good prognosis. However, there may be loss of visual acuity.

Pseudotumour cerebri may be seen in many diseases which can be broadly divided into the following categories:

1. Intracranial venous thrombosis.
2. Endocrine disorders.
    (a) Addison's disease.
    (b) Cushing's disease.
    (c) Hypoparathyroidism.
    (d) Hyper-hypothyroidism.
3. Vitamins and drugs.
    (a) Vitamin A intoxication.
    (b) Iron deficiency.
    (c) Tetracycline therapy.
    (d) Steroid therapy.
    (e) Penicillin therapy.
4. High CSF protein.
    (a) Polyneuritis.
    (b) Tumours of the cauda equina.
5. Haematological.
    (a) Polycythaemia.
    (b) Infectious mononucleosis.
6. (a) Pulmonary encephalopathy.
    (b) Pickwickian syndrome.

7. Miscellaneous.
    (a) Roseola infantum.
    (b) Sydenham's chorea.
    (c) Familial.
8. Idiopathic.

It must be stressed, however, that pseudotumour cerebri is a diagnosis of exclusion in many instances and full investigation of each suspected patient is mandatory.

Further reading

Davis D. O. (1978). Computed tomography of the central nervous system. In *Current Neurology*, Ed. by H. R. Tyler and D. M. Dawson, p. 453. (Boston; Houghton Mifflin Professional Publications)

Houston-Merritt, H. (ed.) (1979). Tumors. In *Textbook of Neurology*, 6th edn. p. 297. (Philadelphia; Lea & Febiger)

Sharpins, W. R. (1972). Intracranial tumors and states causing increased intracranial pressure. In *Textbook of Medicine*, Ed. by J. B. Wyngaarden and L. H. Smith, 3rd edn., p. 2131. (Philadelphia; W. B. Saunders)

Case 35

Answers

1. Giardiasis.
2. (a) Warm-stool microscopy × 3.
    (b) Jejunal intubation for biopsy and juice aspiration.
    (c) Liver function tests.
    (d) Dietary assessment.
    (e) IgE.
    (f) Barium enema.

Discussion

This is a child who has followed a normal course for the first 2 years of his life apart from repeated upper respiratory tract infections which is expected in a child with selective IgA deficiency. With the above history, some diagnoses suggest themselves, such as Hirschsprung's disease, coeliac disease, campylobacter and

Yersinia entercolitis and food allergy. Hirschsprung's disease is unlikely but can be investigated by barium enema, rectal biopsy and anorectal manometry. The infections named above are usually more acute, but chronic problems are sometimes seen. Campylobacter should be isolated from the stool but serological identification is more reliable for Yersinia.

Coeliac disease is unlikely here in view of the normal xylose absorption test and albumin results, lack of steatorrhoea and muscle wasting on examination. However, with a history of failure to thrive, diarrhoea and abdominal pain a jejunal biopsy is always a worthwhile investigation. Food allergy such as cows' milk protein or egg intolerance may present with a similar history but usually this occurs in infancy and not at the age of 4 years.

Giardiasis may be found in 16–21 per cent of children's gastrointestinal tracts. The degree of pathogenicity is still a question. However, there is no doubt that there are three types of presentation: first, acute with foul-smelling stools, flatus, abdominal distension but no blood or pus. Secondly, a subacute infection which may last for some months and can mimic hiatus hernia, cholecystitis and hepatitis. It may be associated with failure to thrive and is probably the category that this child fits into. Thirdly, there is chronic infection lasting for years and associated with malabsorption of fat, D-xylose and vitamin B_{12}, similar to tropical sprue. The question always arises as to why some people are symptomatic and others not. Other factors appear to be at work; those pinpointed are: hypogammaglobulinaemia, deficiency of secretory IgA and unusual bacterial flora of the jejunum which may combine synergistically with giardia to cause symptoms and, lastly, any other pathology present in the patient. The immunoglobulin abnormalities and possibly stasis from constipation might have predisposed this child to giardiasis.

Diagnosis initially should be by microscopy of three warm, concentrated stools. However, the microscopy is positive in only about 30 per cent of patients. Secondly, duodenal intubation with aspiration of jejunal juice may give positive results in about 70 per cent of cases. However, if jejunal biopsy is added approximately 90 per cent of cases will be diagnosed; this is certainly the most reliable investigation.

In this child, lack of weight gain may be due to poor food intake with an inadequate calorie requirement. Thus a dietary assessment should be done. IgE estimation is not a very good indicator of food allergy, but specific IgE to egg, cows' milk and other foodstuffs may be helpful. Liver function tests are indicated in a child who is unwell, especially with a family history of recent infectious hepatitis. Children often have a subclinical form of this infection.

Further reading

Amin, N. (1979). Review. *Postgraduate Medicine*, **66**, 151–162.
Joss, V. and Brueton, M. (1981). Unsuspected giardiasis. *Lancet*, **ii**, 996.
Raizman, R. A. (1976). Giardiasis. An overview for the clinician. *American Journal of Digestive Diseases*, **21**, 1070.
Mandal, B. K. (1981). Intestinal infections in adults and children over the age of two. *Medicine*, Series 4, **2**, 56.
O'Brien, W. (1981). Giardiasis. *Medicine*, Series 4, **4**, 156.

Case 36

Answers

1. In the endocardium of the right ventricle opposite the ventricular septal defect where the jet of blood impinges on the ventricular wall.
2. Long-term antibiotics and removal and replacement of the atrioventricular shunt.

Discussion

This child has signs and symptoms of a chronic infection: lethargy, low-grade pyrexia unresponsive to antibiotics and indicative blood film changes. One negative blood culture does not exclude the diagnosis; a series of blood cultures should be taken when the temperature is spiking. Examination revealed a harsh pansystolic murmur at the left sternal edge, indicative of cardiac pathology; subacute bacterial endorcarditis is therefore a likely diagnosis. Additional corroborative signs are splenomegaly and retinal haemorrhages.

The endocarditis may be secondary to an infected shunt. If not, it will almost certainly have been infected and the value should be replaced after vigorous antibiotic therapy. Infection of the shunt may be confirmed by direct sampling of (CSF) from the valve. Also, complement levels and anti-staphylococcal titres may be raised. The distal catheter may be exteriorized, discarding infected CSF and increasing antibiotic efficiency. The infecting organisms are usually bacterial and of low pathogenicity, initiating sporadic bacteraemias and spiking pyrexias. Mycotic emboli produce ubiquitous vascular lesions, most noticeable in the retina — 'boat-shaped haemorrhage' — and under the nails — 'splinter haemorrhage'. Renal involvement in bacterial endocarditis is due to deposition of immune complexes. Histology reveals a focal proliferative glomerulonephritis with areas of necrosis. Haematuria and proteinuria may be marked. 'Shunt nephritis' following shunt infection is membranoproliferative glomerulonephritis, also probably caused by immune complexes. Again haematuria and proteinuria are induced and the nephrotic syndrome may occur.

All prostheses are susceptible to infection which, once established, is difficult to eradicate as host defences are unable to act synergistically with antibiotics. Prophylactic antibiotics should be given to cover dental and surgical procedures.

Further reading

Cudmore, R. D. and Rickham P. P. (1978). Hydrocephalus. In *Neonatal Surgery*, Ed. by P. P. Rickham, J. Lister and I. M. Irving, 2nd edn., p. 513. (London; Butterworths)
Kin, Y. and Michael, A. F. (1978). Infection and nephritis. In *Pediatric Kidney Disease*, Ed. by C. M. Edelman, p. 828. (Boston; Little, Brown & Co.)

Case 37

Answers

1. Disseminated central nervous system malignancy, particularly non-Hodgkin's lymphoma, leukaemia or neuroblastoma.

Discussion

This boy presents with one of the classic signs of raised intracranial pressure, namely VIth nerve palsy. It is unaccompanied by the symptoms, headache and vomiting. The VIth nerve palsy could be an isolated lesion but there are other signs and symptoms to account for. These are: the upper lip tingling, suggesting involvement of the

Vth nerve sensory nucleus which has a long tail descending to the upper medulla; and the VIIIth nerve deafness with minimal intention tremor on the same side, suggesting a lesion in the cerebellar pontine angle.

The symptoms of later onset are impossible to put down to a posterior fossa lesion. Upper motor neurone signs in the legs with nothing similar in the arms makes a cord lesion involving the motor tracts more likely i.e. anterior, while urinary retention and chest pain may be secondary to root lesions. Thus the signs are best explained by disseminated disease, most likely malignant in the CNS. In children non-Hodgkin's lymphoma and leukaemia may produce such a clinical picture. Early papilloedema may often be present but is not a necessity in such a disseminated picture. Other tumours such as neuroblastoma and rhabdomysarcoma produce neurological signs. Neuroblastoma frequently metastasizes to bone especially the outer table of the skull, causing raised intracranial pressure although cerebral secondaries are rare. Root compression can also be caused by direct extension of the tumour either in the chest or pelvis.

Rhabdomyosarcoma most frequently presents with lesions in the head and neck. A primary in the ear may extend intracerebrally but the tumour does not usually seed through the CSF.

Some primary CNS tumours disseminate via the CSF, namely medulloblastoma and occasionally ependymoma, but these usually present with signs resulting from the primary lesion in the posterior fossa.

Non-Hodgkin's lymphoma arises in lymphatic tissue in 80 per cent of cases, either nodal or extranodal. There is early haematogenous and lymphatic spread, so that the primary site may not always be apparent. The commonest sites for tumour growth are in the head and neck, as an anterior mediastinal mass and in the abdomen with or without intestinal obstruction. Bone pain, marrow infiltration and general symptoms such as fever, weight loss and fatigue may occur. CNS involvement occurs in a significant number of patients, up to one third in some series, with raised intracranial pressure and cranial nerve involvement. Interestingly, leukaemia may result in a similar clinical picture with CNS involvement, since approximately 33 per cent of patients with non-Hodgkin's lymphoma develop leukaemia.

The CT scans were negative, probably because of the diffuse pattern of the malignancy with small deposits low in the posterior fossa, a region difficult to define.

Further reading

Miller, D. R., Pearson, H. A., Baehner, R. L. and Mc Millan, C. W. (eds) (1978). Non-Hodgkin's lymphoma. In *Smith's Blood Diseases of Infancy and Childhood*, pp. 631–637. (St. Louis; C. V. Mosley)
Cooper, I. (1980). Solid tumours of the lymphoid system. *Medicine*, Series 31, **29**, 1493–1500.
Jones, S. E., *et al.* (1973). Non-Hodgkin's lymphomas IV. Clinicopathologic correlation in 405 cases *Cancer*, **31**, 805–823.
Matthews, W. B. and Miller, H. (1972). *Diseases of the Nervous System*, pp. 6–23. (Oxford; Blackwell)
Mott, M. G. (1979). The presentation, management and prognosis of solid tumours in childhood. In *Topics in Paediatrics*. I. *Haematology and Oncology*, Ed. by P. H. Morris Jones, pp. 51–65. (London; Pitman)

Case 38

Answers

1. (a) Vitamin-D resistant rickets (pseudovitamin D deficiency).
   (b) Urinary tract infection.
2. Autosomal recessive.
3. 1-alphahydroxycholecalciferol.

Discussion

When confronted with a case of rickets, the various causes must be systematically considered and excluded one by one. This child does not appear to have been malnourished from the history and, as a regular attender at clinic, probably would have been given vitamin supplementation. Malabsorption certainly is a possibility with mild iron deficiency and a borderline xylose tolerance, but the normal albumin and 3-day faecal fat excretion results make this unlikely. Liver function tests are normal which indicates normal hepatocellular function. Thus hepatic hydroxylation of vitamin D should be intact. If sophisticated laboratory facilities are available 25-OH cholecalciferol can be measured. The next step in the pathway is the kidney. There are several problems that may occur.

First, there are the renal tubular defects, both proximal and distal. In proximal defects there is reduced tubular reabsorption of bicarbonate which is a possibility here in view of the low bicarbonate value with a urinary pH just alkaline. However, there is no hypokalaemia or symptoms from hypercalcuria, both of which occur (Fanconi type of proximal tubular problems is associated with hyperphosphaturia and aminoaciduria, both of which are absent). Distal tubular acidosis occurs because there is poor excretion of titratable acid and NH_4Cl, thus insufficient HCO_3^- is regenerated resulting in insufficient H^+ gradient. This child is able to cope with an acid loading test, putting out an acid urine. Hyperphosphaturia also occurs in hypophosphataemic rickets, in which aminoaciduria does not occur; the condition has an X-linked dominant inheritance. This is unlikely because plasma phosphate is just within the normal range and urinary phosphate output is normal.

Renal hydroxylation of 25-OH cholecalciferol may be defective, either secondary to renal failure (not in this case as the urea result is normal) or in vitamin-D resistant rickets (where the hydroxylation enzyme appears to be missing). If measured, the 25-OH cholecalciferol should be high and the 24-25 dihydroxycholecalciferol may be raised as this pathway is used more frequently if the 1-hydroxylation is blocked. These children generally have low to normal plasma phosphate values and a low calcium level and may present with tetany, aminoaciduria and high alkaline phosphatase activity. This boy does not have all the features, but this is the most likely diagnosis. His parents were first cousins and this fits with the autosomal recessive inheritance of this condition.

Treatment used to be with large doses of vitamin D, but now that 1-α-dihydroxycholecalciferol, the synthetic analogue of 1,25-dihydroxy vitamin D, is available this is usually used especially as it is short acting thus causing less hypercalcaemia. This child also had a urinary tract infection as an incidental finding, but this had no relationship to the original disease.

Further reading

Bricker, N. W., Slatopolsky, E. et al. (1969). Calcium, phosphorous and bone in renal disease and transplant. *Archives of Internal Medicine*, **123**, 543.

Fraser, D. and Scriver, C. R. (1976). Familial forms of vitamin D resistant rickets revisited. *American Journal of Clinical Nutrition*, **29**, 1315.

Leo Laboratories (1977). *One-alpha in the Management of Disorders of Calcium and Phosphorus Metabolism*. (Hayes, Middlesex; Leo Laboratories).

Case 39

Answers

1. (a) Riley–Day syndrome (familial dysautonomia).
   (b) Krabbe's leucodystrophy.
   (c) Perlizaeus–Merzbacher leucodystrophy.
2. (a) Intradermal histamine response.
   (b) Methacholine eye drops.
   (c) Urinary vanillylmandelic acid (VMA) and homomandelic acid (HMA).
   (d) Serum dopamine-β-hydroxylase.
   (e) White cell enzymes.

This child presents with diffuse psychological and physical signs. She exhibits some features of failure to thrive: poor weight gain, irritability with difficult feeding and vomiting. She also displays psychological and neurological signs: temper tantrums with breath-holding episodes (which are normally manifest at 9–12 months) and absent tendon and corneal reflexes, with diminished tear production and corneal ulceration. These signs developed after 4 months of normal life, suggesting either a metabolic or a degenerative disorder. Gut dysfunction alone would not explain the diverse neurological problems.

The combination of impaired sensation (absent corneal reflex) diminished tear production, temper tantrums, smooth tongue (loss of fungiform papillae) and absent tendon reflexes is highly suggestive of Riley–Day syndrome (familial dysautonomia); however, both Krabbe's and Perlizaeus–Merzbacher leucodystrophies may present at this age with highly variable signs. Perlizaeus–Merzbacher disease is less likely as hyperreflexia rather than hyporeflexia obtains.

Postencephalitis syndromes or cerebral sclerosis tend to affect the pyramidal and extrapyramidal systems more than the autonomic and sensory pathways.

Riley–Day syndrome (familial dysautonomia) is a rare, recessively inherited disease, almost exclusively affecting those of eastern European Jewish descent. The infant often has intrauterine growth retardation, but, thereafter, develops normally until 3–6 months when signs develop. Muscle incoordination results in difficulty in deglutition, gagging and aspiration, which, with excess bronchial secretions, produces repeated chest infections, often of sufficient severity to induce cor pulmonale. Excess salivation, causing drooling and hyperhidrosis occur, but tear production is either markedly compromised or absent.

Other autonomic abnormalities include labile hypertension, or orthostatic hypertension, periodic fever and blotching of the skin, especially when excited.

Peripheral sensory dysfunction causes reduction or absence of pain sensation with skin lesions and asymptomatic fractures, absent corneal sensation, taste and deep tendon reflexes.

Histological examination of the peripheral nerve fibres demonstrates reduction both of unmyelinated fibres carrying pain, temperature and taste and of large myelinated fibres carrying afferent impulses from muscle spindles.

Diagnosis is clinical and biochemical. Intradermal histamine produces a much diminished response, methocholine, which detects denervation hypersensitivity of the iris, constricts the pupil within 10 minutes if positive. 25 per cent of the older children lack dopamine-β-hydroxylase which catalyses dopamine to noadrenaline. There is, therefore, a reduction in urinary vanillylmandelic acid (VMA) from noadrenaline metabolism with associated increase in homomandelic acid (HMA) from dopamine.

Treatment is supportive only: treatment of the recurrent chest infections, artificial tears and prevention of injuries. Chlorpromazine has been used with moderate success to control the hypertensive and vomiting episodes. The prognosis is hopeless, death usually occurring in childhood.

The hallmark of Krabbe's leucodystrophy is a rapidly progressive degeneration of the white matter with scattered globoid bodies and myelin balls. Symptoms occur at 4–6 months with implacable crying; this is followed by apathy and stupor. Later the musculature stiffens and eventually becomes totally rigid; gavage is, therefore, necessary for feeding. Deafness, blindness and tonic or clonic fits rapidly supervene. Prognosis is hopeless, death usually occurring within the first year. Just prior to death, musculature becomes flaccid with paralysis.

Perlizaeus–Merzbacher disease is characterized by slow, progressive, universal, symmetrical demyelination of the cerebral white matter, with dense gliosis. The process begins around the ventricles and spreads towards the cortex. Inheritance is either autosomal or sex-linked recessive, but of irregular behaviour. Symptoms become manifest at 3–4 months and are highly variable, but rotary head movements with rotary nystagmus may occur early.

Spasticity occurs first in the legs and then the arms with increased tendon reflexes. The inexorable progression of the disease causes abnormal movements, the weakness and paralysis with subsequent contractures. Although there is no treatment, these patients can experience a normal life span if nursed adequately.

Further reading

Riley-Day syndrome
Ford, F. R. (ed.) (1966). Disorders of the autonomic system. In *Diseases of the Nervous System in Infancy, Childhood and Adolescence*, 5th edn., p. 1190. (Illinois; C. L. Thomas)
Newton, C. F. (1979). Degenerative disease. In *Paediatric Neurology*, Ed. by F. C. Rose, p. 611. (Oxford; Blackwell Scientific Publications)
Paine, R. S. and Oppe, T. E. (eds) (1966). Autonomic function. In *Neurological Examination of Children*, p. 209. (Amsterdam; William Heineman Medical Books)
Krabbe's leucodystrophy
Ford, F. R. (ed.) (1966). Intoxications, metabolic and endocrine disorders. Dietary Deficiencies and allergies involving the nervous system. In *Diseases of the Nervous System in Infancy, Childhood and Adolescence*, 5th edn., p. 757. (Illinois; C. C. Thomas)
Perlizaeus-Merzbacher leucodystrophy
Ford, F. R. (ed.) (1966). Intoxications, metabolic and endocrine disorders. Dietary deficiencies and allergies involving the nervous system. In *Diseases of the Nervous System in Infancy, Childhood and Adolescence*, 5th edn., p. 754. (Illinois; C. C. Thomas)

Case 40

Answers

1. Catheterization.
2. (a) Blood culture.
   (b) Urine culture.
   (c) Full blood count and differential.
   (d) Stool culture.
   (e) Ultrasound.
   (f) Barium enema.
   (g) Indium labelling of WBC with abdominal scan.
3. Pelvic appendix abscess.

Discussion

Initially it appears that this child has a complication of chickenpox, but on closer examination this seems less likely. Chickenpox encephalitis classically starts about 7–10 days after the onset of the rash and affects the cerebellum. To account for the acute retention and constipation, a transverse myelitis would have to be postulated, but the marked pyrexia and second abdominal mass do not fit.

The history given is fairly classic of an acute appendicitis with vomiting, diarrhoea and colicky lower abdominal pain. In a young child, perforation usually occurs early so that the later stage of constipation is not reached. However, this child's condition appears to settle, only to flare up again with a pyrexia, constipation and a dull mass between the bladder and rectum, with secondary acute urinary retention. A pelvic appendix abscess is the most likely diagnosis since it is best felt rectally and the symptoms and signs fit with the duration of the history.

The most important clinical procedure to carry out is relief of the acute urinary retention, most easily done by catheterization. Following this, investigation should be aimed at establishing the diagnosis as far as possible, and ruling out other possibilities. These are: mesenteric adenitis which is usually associated with an upper respiratory tract infection and runs a shorter course; an acute exacerbation of Crohn's disease, unlikely because of the lack of previous symptoms and perianal signs; Hirschsprung's disease or chronic constipation which may cause urinary retention secondary to hard faeces, but again is unlikely with no previous history; urinary tract infection; gastroenteritis, especially *Yersinia enterocolitica*; chronic intussusception which would fit with the earliest symptoms but with no blood per rectum and a mass outside the rectum this is unlikely; lastly, ovarian tumours such as a dermoid which may undergo torsion or become infected and prolapse into the pouch of Douglas.

Investigations such as blood, urine and stool cultures should be done to establish the presence of any pathogens. Full blood count may help to show infection with a high polymorph count of 20.0×10^9. ℓ^{-1} or more, a left shift and toxic granulation. Barium enema should show the position of the caecum and lack of appendix filling. The mass may be delineated by ultrasound, and an indium isotope scan for labelled WBC should show a 'hot spot' over the abscess area. Both the last two investigations have limited availability and laparotomy is the best answer.

Further reading

Homewood-Nixon, H. (1978). *Surgical Conditions in Paediatrics*. Postgraduate Paediatric Series, pp. 188–96. (London; Butterworths)
Black, J. A. (1979). *Paediatric Emergencies*, p. 382. (London; Butterworths)

Case 41

Answers

1. The frontal sinus.
2. (a) Cerebral oedema.
   (b) Superficial venous cerebral thrombosis.
   (c) Extension of the subdural empyema.
3. (a) CT.
   (b) EEG.
   (c) Burr holes.
   (d) Viral titres.

Discussion

This girl demonstrates the classic history of a frontal sinusitis with frontal pain persisting for several days after the resolution of the coryza. The infection then tracked through the skull to produce a subdural empyema. A small collection of pus was drained but this would not explain the gross oedema of the right hemisphere, the papilloedema or the clinical signs. There are non-specific signs of raised intracranial pressure such as the IIIrd and VIth nerve palsies, and specific signs, hemiplegia and hemianopia, which suggest a lesion in the region of the central sulcus. These specific signs could have been caused by gross cerebral oedema, superficial venous thrombophlebitis or extension of the subdural empyema. An extension of the empyema is suggested by her deterioration on the third postoperative day; this was confirmed by a further CT scan. An EEG may be helpful, showing slow wave activity over the lesion; burr holes should reveal a collection of pus. A lumbar puncture is contraindicated although meningeal extension is possible after operative intervention. If necessary CSF should be collected from the cisternae.

Common organisms implicated in subdural empyema are pneumococci, *Streptococcus milleni* and anaerobes. The initial infection may have been local, such as sinusitis or otitis media, or distant as in suppurative lung disease or with a right to left vascular shunt.

Three stages of abscess formation are recognized: first, areas of softening and liquefaction appear; secondly these areas coalesce and pus formation occurs. The final stage is reaction around the abscess, localizing the collection. The clinical signs of a cerebral abscess are extraordinarily varied.

Low-grade infection may produce malaise only, the later signs reflecting a space-occupying lesion. A more virulent infection will produce raised intracranial pressure early with cerebral oedema and focal signs such as hemiplegia and cranial nerve palsies. The CSF is usually sterile, but has raised protein and white cell count, predominantly polymorphonuclear leucocytes.

Treatment is a combination of chemotherapy and surgical drainage where possible. All cases are now potentially curable with prompt diagnosis, but in some series a mortality of 40 per cent still occurs.

Further reading

Harter, D. H. and Merritt, H. H. (1979). Infections. In *A Textbook of Neurology*, Ed. by H. H. Merritt, 6th edn., p. 34. (Philadelphia; Lea and Febiger)
McKinlay, I. A. (1979). Expanding lesions in the head. In *Paediatric Emergencies*, Ed. by J. A. Black, p. 363. (London; Butterworths)
Williams, B. (1982). Subdural empyema. *Hospital Update*, **8**, 111.

Case 42

Answers

1. (a) Sweat test.
   (b) Jejunal biopsy.
   (c) Complement breakdown products after cows' milk challenge.

(d) Stool tryptic activity.
   (e) Stool culture.
   (f) Stool and urine reducing substances.
   (g) Lactose tolerance.
   (h) D-xylose absorption test.
2. (a) Cystic fibrosis.
   (b) Coeliac disease.
   (c) Cows' milk protein intolerance.
   (d) Lactose intolerance.
   (e) Gastroenteritis.

Discussion

The most likely diagnosis in this child is cystic fibrosis. He has had abnormal stools since birth, he is failing to thrive and has a raised respiratory rate and persitent substernal recession. These last two signs, with overexpansion, are often the earliest signs of chest involvement occurring before any radiological changes. A paroxysmal cough culminating in vomiting is characteristic of cystic fibrosis. A similar situation obtains in pertussis, but this child has had two triple immunizations, which reduces the likelihood of pertussis considerably.

Cystic fibrosis is the commonest inherited disease in England, occurring in approximately 1 in 2000 births with a carrier rate of 1 in 20–30. There is, however, a high spontaneous mutation rate. Cystic fibrosis may be diagnosed *in utero* if the fetus has suffered meconium peritonitis with subsequent peritoneal calcification. This would be detected on X-ray should there be maternal indications. Recently it has been demonstrated that amniotic fluid from fetuses with cystic fibrosis is significantly deficient in methylumbelliferyl-guanidinebenzoate (MUGB) reactive proteases. In a small study in the USA it has been possible to diagnose intrauterine cystic fibrosis reliably. In the neonatal period the first meconium passed can be tested for albumin which is present in cystic fibrosis; however, there is a high incidence both of false-positive and of false-negative results.

The neonate may present with meconium ileus, requiring either a Gastrografin enema or laparotomy.

The sweat test is a useful screening test if at least 100 mg of sweat is collected. A sodium concentration of greater than 60 mmol. ℓ^{-1} is diagnostic, and values between 40 and 60 mmol. ℓ^{-1} necessitate a repeat examination. Other causes of a high sweat sodium concentration include Addison's disease, congenital adrenal hyperplasia, nephrogenic diabetes insipidus, glucose-6-phosphatase deficiency, fucosidosis and ectodermal dysplasia with hypoparathyroidism and sensori-neural deafness.

Treatment of cystic fibrosis is by replacing the deficient pancreatic enzymes and treating all chest complications vigorously with physiotherapy and antibiotics, which may be administered by aerosol as well as systemically. However, cor pulmonale secondary to lung parenchymal damage is still a major cause of death.

This child also received cereals, containing gluten, and cows' milk. Therefore, coeliac disease and cows' milk protein intolerance must be excluded. Children with coeliac disease often have a hypochromic microcytic anaemia secondary to iron deficiency but this would not be manifest at 9 months. Folate deficiency also occurs and a macrocytic blood film may occur when the iron deficiency is corrected. Diagnosis may be confirmed by duodenal or jejunal mucosal biopsy, demonstrating abnormal histology, followed by remission of symptoms when gluten is excluded from the diet.

There is a stunting or flattening of the villi and deepening of the crypts and a cellular infiltrate consisting of eosinophils and lymphocytes, with an increased number of IgM secreting cells. These changes should revert to normal on a gluten-free diet. If the diagnosis remains in doubt after jejunal biopsy and the symptoms remain, the child should be placed on a gluten-free diet, have a repeat jejunal biopsy and then be subjected to a gluten challenge to determine the effect of gluten on the small-bowel mucosa.

The diagnosis of cows' milk protein enteropathy may be difficult to substantiate. The history may be suggestive with the onset of symptoms coinciding with the introduction of cows' milk. Jejunal mucosal damage is patchy and normal mucosa may be biopsied; double port capsules have been introduced to circumvent this problem. There are no specific histological changes in cows' milk protein enteropathy, and microscopy may reveal a non-specific partial villous atrophy. A rise in complement breakdown products following a cows' milk challenge is supportive. Recently, however, this has been questioned. Often the diagnosis is made clinically following dietary exclusion of cows' milk protein.

Lactose intolerance is commonly secondary to mucosal damage induced by gastroenteritis; primary lactose intolerance is rare. The clinical response to an oral load of lactose is of prime importance in the diagnosis; supportive evidence may be gained from a lactose tolerance test. A rise in blood glucose of less than 1.1 mmol. ℓ^{-1} is suggestive of lactose deficiency; however, false positives can occur. Alternatively, the hydrogen breath test can be used, demonstrating a rise in end expiratory hydrogen concentration after lactose ingestion.

Decreased xylose absorption implies small-bowel brush-border damage, but is of little value in differentiating the causes of an enteropathy.

Further reading

Anderson, C. M. and Goodchild, M. C. (eds) (1976). Cystic fibrosis. In *Manual of Diagnosis and Management*, (Oxford; Blackwell)
Katz, A. J. and Falchuk, E. M. (1975). Current concepts in gluten sensitive enteropathy (coeliac sprue). *Pediatric Clinics of North America*, **22**, 767.
Lebenthal, E. (1975). Cows' milk protein allergy. *Pediatric Clinics of North America*, **22**, 827.
Lebenthal, E. (1975). Small intestinal dissacharidase deficiencies. *Pediatric Clinics of North America*, **22**, 757.
Shwachman, H. (1975). Gastrointestinal manifestations of cystic fibrosis. *Pediatric Clinics of North America*, **22**, 787.

Case 43

Answers

1. Serum level of carbamazepine.
2. Deliberate ingestion of carbamazepine.

Discussion

The initial presentation of this child could suggest a migrainous episode. She had a headache, dizziness, visual disturbances and vomiting. However, the visual disturbances of migraine are usually described as flashing lights followed by bilateral scotomata; diplopia is rare, and slow pupillary reflexes are also not a feature of migraine. Ataxic gait and limb weakness may occur but the neurological symptoms usually develop rapidly and then remit equally rapidly, often within an hour, leaving the patient with a unilateral throbbing headache.

She had had a previous episode, also of short duration, some months earlier, also with no neurological sequelae. This militates against intracranial pathology, such as a space-occupying lesion or vascular accident. Central nervous system infection is similarly unlikely. Two drugs are mentioned. Insulin overdose, with hypoglycaemic symptoms such as sweating, tachycardia, ataxia and tremor, is unlikely as she is still experiencing severe symptoms with a normal blood glucose level. The most likely diagnosis is, therefore, carbamazepine toxicity. Carbamazepine is structurally related to the tricyclic antidepressants and its toxic effects are similar. Toxic effects include headache, dizziness, drowsiness, diplopia, blurred vision, ataxia and gastrointestinal disturbance. Cardiovascular effects include hypertension, hypotension and ectopic beats. Rarer toxic effects include morbilliform skin rashes, Stevens–Johnson syndrome, bone-marrow depression, jaundice and renal failure.

This child later admitted taking her father's tablets deliberately before both episodes. The psychodynamics of suicide attempts are multiple and complex, but some attempts are related to specific occurrences. In this instance, the vulval bruising noted in the examination was the result of a sexual advance by the child's father.

Further reading

Adams, R. D. (1977). Headache. In *Harrison's Principles of Internal Medicine*, Ed. by G. W. Thorn, R. D. Adams, E. Braunwald, K. J. Isselbacher, R. G. Petersdorf, 8th edn., p. 22. (New York; McGraw Hill)
Congdon, P. J. (1979). Migraine in childhood, a review. *Clinical Pediatrics*, **18**, 353.
Eisenburg, L. (1980). Adolescent suicide. *Pediatrics*, **66**, 696.
Henderson, D. J. (1975). Normal and abnormal human sexuality. In *Comprehensive Textbook of Psychiatry*, Ed. by A. M. Freedman, H. I. Kaplan, B. J. Sadock, 2nd edn., p. 1530. (Baltimore; Williams and Wilkins)
Nakashima, I. L. (1977). Incest: review and clinical experience. *Pediatrics*, **60**, 696.
Schneidman, E. S. (1975). Adolescent suicide. In *Comprehensive Textbook of Psychiatry*, Ed. by A. M. Freedman, H. I. Kaplan and B. J. Sadock, 2nd edn., p. 1774. (Baltimore; Williams and Wilkins)
Wade, A. (ed.) (1977). Phenytoin and other anticonvulsants. In *Martindale. The Extra Pharmacopoeia*, 27th edn., p. 1236. (London; Pharmaceutical Press)

Case 44

Answers

1. (a) Crohn's disease.
   (b) Tuberculous ileitis.

2. (a) Barium enema.
    (b) Colonoscopy.
    (c) Mucosal biopsy.
    (d) Mantoux test.
    (e) Chest X-ray.
    (f) Stool culture.

Discussion

The presence of a spontaneous perianal fistula, as evidenced by soiling of the underwear without incontinence, suggests Crohn's disease, or, more rarely, tuberculous ileitis as possible diagnoses. Other compatible features include unaltered blood mixed with watery semi-solid stools, weight loss and a painful abdominal mass without tenesmus. Tenesmus is common in ulcerative colitis, whilst spontaneous fistulae are rare. Tuberculous enteritis and fistula-*in-ano* formation are rare in childhood and usually occur in children with suppurative pulmonary tuberculosis, who then swallow the infected sputum. This child had no pulmonary symptoms, but it is a diagnosis to consider in the debilitated child.

Infective causes of bloody diarrhoea such as Shigella and Campylobacter infestation should be excluded by repeated stool cultures. Intestinal mucosal infarctions during a sickling crisis causes rectal bleeding. However, such episodes are accompanied by a fall in Hb level and severe abdominal pain with bleeding occurring after some days, then resolving spontaneously.

Rectal bleeding is uncommon in paediatrics and should always be investigated thoroughly. Upper intestinal bleeding, unless catastrophic, will produce malaena. Causes of frank rectal bleeding include bleeding diatheses, inflammatory bowel diseases and local causes such as rectal prolapse or fissure-*in-ano*. Common surgical causes are duplication cysts, volvulus and intussusception. Rarely, polyps, haemorrhoids or neoplasms may present with rectal bleeding in paediatric practice.

Further reading

Dyer, N. H. (1975). Chronic inflammatory disorders. In *Paediatric Gastroenterology*, Ed. by C. M. Anderson and V. Burke, pp. 411, 453. (Oxford; Blackwell Scientific Publications)

Lorber, J. (1978). Diseases due to infection. In *Textbook of Paediatrics*, Ed. by J. O. Forfar and G. C. Arneil, 2nd edn., p. 1222. (London; Churchill Livingstone)

Spitz, L. (1979). Acute abdominal emergencies. In *Paediatric Emergencies*, Ed. by J. A. Black, p. 386. (London; Butterworths)

Case 45

Answers

1. Inhalation of a foreign body.
2. Bronchoscopy.

Discussion

Inhalation of a foreign body in a child is particularly common under the age of 4 years. Peanuts and other edible nuts comprise about 50 per cent of inhaled foreign bodies; this child inhaled a pistachio nut! The problem is fairly easy to diagnose if there is a history of inhalation followed by the onset of cough and wheeze. This is usually caused by the initial irritation following a foreign body in the airways with choking and coughing; mucosal oedema then may result from chemical irritation due to nut oils, often arachidonic acid. This may cuase some wheeze, but wheeze also results from an obstructive hyperinflation of part or all of one lung, where the foreign body acts as a ball valve allowing air in but not out. However, a collapse may occur distal to the foreign body and this can become secondarily infected.

Delay in diagnosis occurs in about a third of cases. About 40 per cent of these are due to the fact that the parents are unaware that the child has inhaled anything as in the above case. However, attention should have been paid earlier to the fact that this girl had a cough for 3 days without a temperature or preceding coryza, followed by a severe illness with a small segmental collapse/consolidation which did not improve rapidly. Partially treated meningitis was then a complicating feature, probably from persisting septicaemia secondary to the chest infection. Hyperinflation of the left lung is an unusual feature at this stage but possibly resulted from movement of the impacted nut while coughing. Generally the clinical picture associated with an unknown retained foreign body follows various patterns, wheezy bronchitis, failed resolution of an acute respiratory infection, chronic cough with haemoptysis, chronic cough and lung collapse and respiratory failure. If a child presents with a first attack of wheezy bronchitis this diagnosis should be borne in mind, but when there is a previous history of wheezing, as in this little girl, the problem is all the more difficult.

Any foreign body must be removed. Generally this is done by

bronchoscopy but if the material is embedded in the bronchial wall, a segment or lobe may need to be removed. This, of course, should be preceded by a bronchoscopy.

Further reading

Rothman, B. F., *et al*. (1980). Foreign bodies in the larynx and tracheo-bronchial tree in children. A review of 225 cases. Annals of Otology, Rhinology and Laryngology, **89**, 434–436.
Williams, H. E. and Phelan, P. D. (eds.) (1975). Pulmonary complications of inhalation. In *Respiratory Illness in Children*, pp. 237–60. (Oxford; Blackwell Scientific Publications)

Case 46

Answers

1. (a) Toxocara fluorescent antibody.
   (b) Toxocara skin test.
   (c) Immunoglobulins.
   (d) Ascaris complement fixation.
2. (a) *Toxocara canis* infestation.
   (b) Ascaris species (rare).

Discussion

The most striking investigative abnormality in this child is the absolute eosinophilia. Causes of eosinophilia include allergic reactions, parasitic infestation, drugs such as penicillin and streptomycin, skin diseases (including psoriasis and pemphigus), pulmonary eosinophilia, Hodgkin's disease, eosinophilic leukaemia and polyarteritis nodosa. The length of history and lack of any systemic physical findings make malignancy unlikely and this degree of eosinophilia is particularly seen in parasitic infestations or pulmonary eosinophilia.

Pulmonary eosinophilia is classified by aetiology. Löffler's syndrome or simple pulmonary eosinophilia is probably a hypersensitivity reaction to a multitude of agents including drugs, inhaled allergens and desensitizing vaccines. Pulmonary eosinophilia occurs in a small percentage of asthmatics. The aetiology is unknown, but again may be a hypersensitivity reaction. Chest X-ray reveals patchy shadowing.

Tropical eosinophilia is similar to Löffler's syndrome but caused by the migrating larvae of filarial worms. Visceral larva migrans caused by *Toxocara canis* produces a similar syndrome in temperate climates.

The diagnosis that most closely fits with the findings in this boy of eosinophilia and an occular mass is visceral larva migrans caused by the larvae of *Toxocara canis*. The role of *T. catis* in visceral larva migrans is still not determined.

Puppies are the main domestic carriers of *T. canis* and there is orofaecal spread to humans. The soil in many parklands and waste areas contains viable toxocara eggs which can be ingested by children. The eggs hatch in the intestine and the larvae migrate randomly through the body and may encyst in any organ. The younger child usually has systemic signs and symptoms such as pyrexia, pica, failure to thrive, anaemia and hepatosplenomegaly. Involvement of the lung produces cough and wheezing. Neurological involvement may cause bizarre peripheral signs, fits or coma. In the older child it is not uncommon for the eye alone to be affected, with no other physical findings. Asymptomatic siblings of affected children are occasionally shown to have hepatomegaly and eosinophilia. Certain diagnosis can be gained only by biopsy, but the indirect fluorescent antibody test and toxocara skin test are becoming more reliable. Both serology and skin test may be negative if the infection is confined to the eye. Treatment of visceral larva migrans is with diethylcarbamazine or thiobendazole.

The larvae of certain other worms are capable of causing visceral larva migrans. Such worms include *Ascaris suum* from pigs and, rarely, *Ascaris lumbricoides*. Again, intense eosinophilia is seen, but it is extremely rare to have a single ocular granulomatous lesion with no other manifestations.

Further reading

Jelliffe, D. B. and Jelliffe, E. F. P. (1978). In *Diseases of Children in the Subtropics and Tropics*, Ed. by D. B. Jelliffe, S. Paget and J. Stanfield, 3rd edn., p. 515. (London; Edward Arnold)

Raistrick, E. R. (1975). Adult toxocaral infection with focal retinal lesions. *British Medical Journal*, **iii**, 416.

Raistrick, E. R. (1976). Ocular toxocariasis in adults, *British Journal of Ophthalmology*, **60**, 365.

Zyngier, F. R. (1976). Toxocariasis and ascariasis: a comparison. I. Description of infection, haematological response, serum proteins and skin test with *Toxocara canis* antigen. *Revista do Instituto de Medicina Tropical de Sao Paulo*, **18**, 251.

Zyngier, F. R. (1976). Ascariasis and toxocariasis. II. Difficulties in the differential serological diagnosis employing a *Toxocara canis* antigen. *Revista do Instituto de Medicina Tropical de Sao Paulo*, **18**, 427.

Case 47

Answers

1. Fanconi syndrome.
2. Cystinosis.
3. (a) Urinary amino acids.
   (b) Slit lamp examination of the eye.
   (c) Bone marrow aspiration.
   (d) Lymph node biopsy.
   (e) Sodium bicarbonate loading either by infusion or orally.
   (f) Urinary phosphate excretion.
   (g) Urinary potassium.
4. (a) Potassium supplementation.
   (b) Correction of acidosis with citrate solution and/or sodium bicarbonate.
   (c) Vitamin D supplements or an analogue such as 1 α-cholecalciferol.
   (d) Sufficient fluid intake.
   (e) Hydrochlorothiazide.
5. (a) Heavy metal poisoning, e.g. lead.
   (b) Hereditary fructose intolerance.
   (c) Tyrosinosis.
   (d) Wilson's disease.
   (e) Galactosaemia.

Discussion

This child presents a classic picture of Fanconi syndrome: a normal child at birth developing growth failure with rickets, constipation and finally an acute illness secondary to renal pathology. Fanconi syndrome consists of renal tubular acidosis affecting the proximal tubules, together with aminoaciduria, glycosuria, hyperphosphaturia and hypokalaemia.

In proximal renal tubular acidosis (PTA) there is reduced reabsorption of bicarbonate even with a mild acidosis present (i.e. HCO_3^-, 16–22 mmol ℓ^{-1}). Below this bicarbonate level there are sufficient hydrogen ions secreted by the proximal tubule to reabsorb bicarbonate. Distal tubular function is intact, thus in a case such as this the urinary pH is appropriately acidic, unlike distal tubular acidosis where an alkaline urine is found despite a metabolic acidosis.

In normal patients the bicarbonate renal threshold is 24–26 mmol. ℓ^{-1}. Sodium bicarbonate supplements in the order of 5–15 mmol. kg^{-1}. 24 h can be given in PTA for maintenance but generally a mixture of sodium and potassium citrate is given which corrects the acidosis and electrolyte deficits.

Potassium is lost both from proximal and from distal tubules resulting in severe weakness, thus large amounts of potassium — usually in the citrate mixture as described above — are given as maintenance once the initial deficit has been corrected. Hypokalaemia plus tubular damage occurring as a result of the cystinosis can impair the ability to concentrate the urine. Thus diarrhoea and vomiting result in very rapid dehydration and acidosis. These episodes can cause episodic fever.

Hyperphosphaturia results in hypophosphataemia initially, and only as renal function fails does the serum phosphate level rise. Hypercalcuria occurs but secondary hyperparathyroidism maintains a normal serum calcium at the expense of the bones which become demineralized causing rickets or osteomalacia. Vitamin D is given but there is resistance to several of the effects. However, large doses may improve calcium absorption and partially restore tubular transport of amino acids, glucose and phosphate. Intestinal absorption of calcium is not always depressed in multiple tubular dysfunction; thus calcium supplements are only sometimes required. The vitamin D analogue 1 α-cholecalciferol may prove to be more appropriate medication since it bypasses the kidney hydroxylation of vitamin D to its active metabolite, 1, 25-dihydroxycholecalciferol.

Cystinosis is the most likely diagnosis since the parents were first cousins and the family history is in favour of an autosomal recessive inheritance. Cystine crystals are most readily demonstrated in the cornea by slit lamp examination, also in bone marrow aspirates. At a later stage the cornea becomes cloudy. Deposits are also found in the rest of the reticuloendothelial system, i.e. liver, spleen and lymph nodes, and may be seen in biopsy material.

Hydrochlorothiazide given for maintenance therapy may facilitate the correction of acidosis and healing of rickets by increasing proximal tubular absorption of sodium, bicarbonate, phosphate and calcium. In turn this should reduce the solute load in the urine and thus the degree of polyuria. Fluid intake must always be great enough to balance the obligatory polyuria.

Further reading

Brodehl, J. (1978). The Fanconi syndrome. In *Paediatric Kidney Disease*, Ed. by C. N. Edelmann, p. 81. (Boston; Little Brown)
Schneider, J. A. Cystinosis and the Fanconi syndrome. In *The Metabolic Basis of Inherited Disease*, p. 670. (New York; McGraw Hill)

Case 48

Answers

1. Acute intermittent porphyria.
2. Autosomal dominant.

Discussion

The behaviour of the child after parental separation had been appropriate, if unreasonable. However, there had been a recent behavioural change with inappropriate responses, usually associated with abdominal pain. During one such attack — probably precipitated by otitis media, — hyponatraemia, leucocytosis, hypertension, pigmentation and a loss of deep tendon reflexes were observed. These findings are consistent with acute intermittent porphyria. Porphyria variegata differs clinically in the skin manifestations which include a photosensitive rash with blistering and cicatrization. Temporal lobe epilepsy had been excluded by an EEG and a trial of carbamazepine. Many aspects of this case are seen in chronic lead intoxication, but not hyponatraemia, uraemia, a normal Hb level and pigmentation. The recurrent nature of the episodes is also not characterisitic.

Porphyria is a rare disease, subdivided into three groups: erythropoietic, erythrohepatic and hepatic. Acute intermittent porphyria and porphyria variegata are hepatic variants. Inheritance of both is autosomal dominant and attacks, which may last from hours to weeks, occur after puberty, more commonly in females. Episodes may be precipitated by drugs such as barbiturates, sulphonamides and griseofulvin, hormones such as oestrogens, infection and dieting. Abdominal symptoms include localized or generalized pain variably accompanied by vomiting and constipation; neurological symptoms are more varied and range from personality changes and mild neurological deficits to quadriplegia and death from respiratory paralysis. Skin manifestations are usually confined to pigmentation without blistering in areas exposed to sunlight. Biochemical abnormalities include hyponatraemia and uraemia, and less commonly hypokalaemia and hypochloraemia. Diagnosis is confirmed by detecting elevated levels of porphyrin precursors in the urine and faeces. In acute intermittent porphyria δ-aminolevulinic acid and porphobilinogen are markedly increased in the urine and coproporphyrinogen and uroporphyrinogen in the faeces are either normal or slightly increased. In porphyria variegata, the urinary findings are similar but there is a marked increase in faecal porphyrins. Lead poisoning can be differentiated by a normal porphobilinogen and raised δ-aminolevulinic acid level.

Erythrocyte levels of uroporphyrinogen-1-synthetase may be reduced in acute intermittent porphyria but this is an unreliable indication.

Urinary coproporphyrinogen may be increased in liver disease; ulcerative lesions of upper gastrointestinal tract may produce increased faecal porphyrins from denaturation of Hb.

Treatment is by avoiding precipitating factors as far as possible and correcting electrolyte imbalance during the episode.

Further reading

Marver, H. S. and Schmid, R. (1972). The porphyrias. In *The Metabolic Basis of Inherited Disease*, Ed. by J. B. Stanbury, J. B. Wyngaarden and D. S. Fredrickson, 3rd edn., p. 1087. (New York; McGraw-Hill)

Tschundy, D. P. (1979). Porphyrias. In *Chemical Diagnosis of Disease*, Ed. by S. S. Brown, F. L. Mitchell and D. S. Young, p. 1039. (Amsterdam; Elsevier North — Holland Biochemical Press)

Yi Yung Hsia, D. (ed.) (1966). *The Porphyrias*. In *Inborn Errors of Metabolism*, 2nd edn. p. 333. (Chicago; Year Book Medical Publishers)

Case 49

Answers

1. (a) Pyloric stenosis.
   (b) Hiatus hernia or gastro-oesophageal reflux.
   (c) Cows' milk intolerance.
   (d) Inborn error of metabolism: organic aciduria.
   (e) Raised intracranial pressure.
2. (a) Test feed.
   (b) Barium swallow and follow-through.
   (c) pH and calculation of anion gap.
   (d) Urinary and plasma amino acid profile.
   (e) Blood ammonia.
   (f) Blood lactic acid level.
   (g) Jejunal biopsy.
   (h) RAST — specific IgE for cows' milk.
   (i) CT scan.

Discussion

This child presents with a classic history of pyloric stenosis, in a form not seen so frequently today. Pyloric stenosis should always be considered in a previously healthy baby, particularly a boy, aged 1–3 months, who has significant vomiting. Five times as many cases occur in male than in female infants. The onset often occurs in the second or third week with non-projectile vomiting, which proceeds to projectile vomiting, either after every feed or intermittently. The infant is usually hungry and is anxious to take another feed immediately. Sometimes the baby becomes lethargic, as in this case, and only small volumes of feed are taken. With such poor intake and incomplete pyloric obstruction, little or no vomiting occurs, but there is gross weight loss. Full-volume tube feeds result in marked vomiting and visible gastric peristalsis. With recurrent vomiting, hypochloraemic alkalosis, variable dehydration and sodium and potassium losses occur. To try to prove pyloric stenosis a test feed is generally given, first to see gastric peristalsis and secondly to feel the pyloric tumour. A barium meal can be carried out if the test feed is inconclusive. This will show delayed gastric emptying and the 'string sign' of the pylorus.

Differential diagnosis of cows' milk intolerance, hiatus hernia or gastro-oesophageal reflux are possible. Hiatus hernia or gastro-oesophageal reflux do not generally cause marked metabolic abnormalities and the history usually starts from shortly after birth. Reluctance to feed is very unusual, but failure to thrive is common. Diagnosis should be by barium swallow.

Cows' milk intolerance often presents with a history of reluctance to take feeds and vomiting, but frequently there are other symptoms such as diarrhoea, rash, wheezing and blood in the stools, not present in this case. A jejunal biopsy would show a non-specific small-bowel enteropathy. Serial biopsies following a milk-free diet and subsequent cows' milk challenge are the best method of diagnosis. Specific IgE for cows' milk does not correspond well with clinical status.

Unexplained acidosis with an anion gap exceeding 16 mmol. ℓ^{-1} is associated with abnormal levels of ketones, salicylates, lactate or organic acids. Proprionic acidaemia and methylmalonic acidaemia (organic acidurias) usually present with disease early in life, but occasionally presentation is delayed up to the age of 3 months. Failure to thrive, with vomiting and marked intolerance to the usualy dietary intake of protein, are the presenting symptoms. There can also be episodes of acute illness heralded by ketonuria. This is followed by vomiting which may be so severe that it suggests the presence of pyloric stenosis. Hyperglycinaemia may be present together with other raised amino acid levels in the blood, and sometimes aminoaciduria. Hyperammonaemia can be found in both organic acidurias and with defects of the enzymes of the urea cycle. In the latter progressive lethargy commonly developes within the first 48 hours of life. This may be associated with jerky movements or frank seizures, before progressing to deep coma. This case has many features of methylmalonic acidaemia but the raised HCO_3^- value suggests alkalosis rather than acidosis. Lactic acidosis is unlikely for the same reason, and most cases have marked signs by the age of 3 months.

Inborn errors of carbohydrate metabolism are unlikely to present at the age of 2–3 months. Reducing substances should be present in the urine, and clinical features of hepatomegaly, jaundice, cataracts, irritability and convulsions may be marked at this stage.

Lastly, alteration of behaviour with vomiting and lethargy should always suggest an intracranial lesion. A CT scan should assist diagnosis.

Further reading

Anderson, C. M. and Blackwell, V. (eds) (1975). Gastrointestinal manifestations of intolerance or allergy to milk protein. Hiatal hernia. In *Paediatric Gastroenterology*, pp. 225–230, 508–515. (Oxford; Blackwell)
Nixon, H. H. (ed.) (1978) Infantile hypertrophic pyloric stenosis, In *Surgical Conditions in Paediatrics, pp. 139–145. (London; Butterworths)*
Nyhan, W. L. (1980). *Inherited Metabolic Disease.*
Sinclar, L. (ed.) (1980). Disorders of intermediary metabolism. In *Metabolic Disease in Childhood, pp. 334–362. (Oxford; Blackwell Scientific Publications)*

Case 50

Answers

1. (a) Galactosaemia.
   (b) Fructosaemia.
   (c) Neonatal hepatitis.
   (d) Sepsis.
2. (a) Conjugated and unconjugated bilirubin.
   (b) Blood cultures.
   (c) Analysis of the reducing substance.
   (d) Urinalysis for protein and amino acids.
   (e) Enzyme levels.

Discussion

The presenting clinical sign in this child is prolonged jaundice, the causes of which are protean. It is diagnostically useful, therefore, to determine the relative amounts of conjugated and unconjugated bilirubin. Further positive signs are vomiting with non-bloody diarrhoea, hepatomegaly and poor weight gain. Positive laboratory data include hypoglycaemia, with reducing substances in the urine, prolonged PTT/KCT, and a metabolic acidosis associated with a neutral urinary pH, suggesting a tubular defect in hydrogenon homeostasis. Those features are compatible with galactosaemia and fructosaemia; the infant must have previously ingested the relevant sugar. However, some other diagnoses to exclude are neonatal hepatitis, sepsis and Fanconi's syndrome. Neonatal hepatitis, unlike cirrhosis, is not associated with renal abnormalities, but it may be associated with hypoglycaemia secondary to the compromised liver. Galactosuria may occur as the insulted liver is unable to metabolize galactose rapidly, resulting in urinary excretion.

Sepsis may cause hypoglycaemia, a metabolic acidosis, which is combined with an acid urine and unconjugated hyperbilirubinaemia. It is not associated with galactosuria but should, nevertheless, be excluded. Fanconi's syndrome, which produces renal tubular acidosis, is not associated with jaundice, and hypoglycaemia is rare, despite glycosuria.

Galactosaemia is a rare, recessively inherited disease occurring in between 1 in 30 000 to 1 in 70 000 live births. Two types occur related to different enzyme defects. Galactokinase deficiency is associated with cataract formation only; galactose-1-phosphate uridyl transferase deficiency causes multi-system involvement of widely varying severity. The mild Duarte variant causes no symptoms but erythrocyte galactose-1-phosphate uridyl transferase activity is reduced. The more severe forms present a few days after the ingestion of lactose.

Prolonged jaundice is often the presenting sign. Diarrhoea and vomiting, hepatomegaly and failure to thrive follow rapidly. Cataracts may occur in the first few days of life, but are visible with a slit lamp only as they consist of small punctate lesions in the fetal lens nucleus. Hypoglycaemia, secondary to galactose ingestion, is caused by the inhibition of phosphoglucomutase and glucose-6-phosphatase by galactose-1-phosphate. Hepatic damage causes hepatomegaly, jaundice, hypoproteinaemia and hypoprothrombinaemia. Early biopsy reveals fatty infiltration, fibrosis, bile duct proliferation and a characteristic pseudoalveolar arrangement of hepatic cells. Later macronodular cirrhosis supervenes. Renal accumulation of galactose-1-phosphate induces proximal tubular acidosis, phosphaturia, bicarbonaturia producing acidosis, proteinuria and generalized aminoaciduria. The aminoaciduria is non-specific, but there is a predominance of the neutral dibasic acids serine, glycine, alanine, threonine, glutamine and valine. The phosphaturia may cause rickets. Rarely, pseudotumour cerebri occurs secondary to diffuse cerebral oedema.

Treatment consists of a lactose-free diet, for example Nutramigen. Therapeutic efficacy is followed by serial measurements of erythrocyte galactose-1-phosphate level.

Fructosaemia is an equally rare autosomal recessively inherited disease with an incidence of approximately 1 in 40 000 live births. Two varieties occur: fructokinase deficiency which causes benign fructosuria only and the more severe fructose-1-phosphate aldolase deficiency with accumulation of fructose-1-phosphate in many tissues which causes widespread systemic effects.

There are three aldolase isoenzymes: A in muscle, B in liver and C in the brain; in this disease the liver isoenzyme is deficient.

Clinical presentation of fructose-1-phosphate aldolase deficiency varies with age. In the infant, severe hypoglycaemia is induced 20–30 minutes after ingestion of fructose, accompanied by sweating, irritability, vomiting and possibly convulsions with loss of consciousness. If the diagnosis is missed, chronic fructose poisoning causes jaundice, fatty infiltration of the liver, hepatomegaly and hepatocyte cytoplasmic dissolution; eventually cirrhosis supervenes with ascites and oedema. The vomiting worsens in frequency and severity and the child fails to thrive. Accumulation of fructose-1-phosphate in the kidney produces a proximal tubular acidosis, phosphaturia, proteinuria and aminoaciduria.

In the older child, hypoglycaemia is normally not a feature, but shortly after ingestion of fructose severe epigastric pain is experienced, followed by nausea and vomiting.

Diagnosis is confirmed by detecting fructosaemia, hyperbilirubinaemia, hypophosphataemia, raised free fatty acids and raised liver enzymes. Fructosuria, phosphaturia, proteinuria and aminoaciduria occur. Fructose tolerance tests should be performed with extreme care, if at all, as profound hypoglycaemia, sufficient to cause neurological damage, may occur.

Treatment is a fructose-free diet and the prognosis is generally good; however, a more guarded opinion must be given in the more severe cases.

Further reading

Froesch, E. R. (1972). Essential fructosuria and hereditary fructose intolerance. In *The Metabolic Basis of Inherited Disease*, Ed. by J. B. Stanbury, H. B. Wyngaarden and D. S. Fredrickson, 3rd edn., p. 131. (New York; McGraw-Hill)

Gitzelman, R. and Hansen, R. G. (1979). Galactose metabolism, hereditary defects and their clinical significance. In *Inherited Disorders of Carbohydrate Metabolism*, Ed. by D. Burman, J. B. Holton and C. A. Pennock, p. 61. (Lancaster; MTP Press)

Segal, S. (1972). Disorders of galactose metabolism. In *The Metabolic Basis of Inherited Disease*, Ed. by J. B. Stanbury, J. B. Wyngaarden and D. S. Fredrickson, 3rd edn., (New York; McGraw-Hill)

Case 51

Answers

1. (a) Dermatomyositis.
   (b) Polymyositis.
   (c) Viral infection.
   (d) Limb girdle muscular dystrophy.
2. (a) Creatinine phosphokinase.
   (b) Electromyogram (EMG).
   (c) Muscle biopsy.
   (d) Anti-nuclear factor.
   (e) Bone marrow aspiration.
   (f) Viral studies.
3. (a) Collodion patches.
   (b) Calcinotic nodules.
   (c) Telangiectasia on eyelids and nailbeds.
   (d) Retinitis.
   (e) Pulmonary manifestations.
   (f) Abdominal pain.
   (g) Haematemesis and malaena from ulceration.

Discussion

Dermatomyositis is usually diagnosed on the clinical features of symmetrical weakness of limb girdle muscles and typical skin rashes and confirmed by elevation of serum muscle enzyme activities, an abnormal EMG and muscle biopsy samples showing inflammatory myositis. Dermatomyositis in childhood has been recorded in association with leukaemia and hypogammaglobulinaemia. These children are said to get gradual thickening and hardening of the muscles with an atypical rash. There are two features that separate dermatomyositis in childhood from that seen in adults. First, the presence of vasculitis; and secondly the late development of calcinosis.

The above case exhibits only some of the typical features with fever, pain, weight loss, general malaise, peripheral oedema of the hands and feet, typical facial rash especially in the periorbital area and forehead. The rash may extend to the neck, shoulders, upper chest, extensor surfaces and front of legs. There may be red patches over bony prominences, such as the knuckles, which can flake and are then called collodion patches; ulceration in the skin folds; telangiectasia around the nail beds; mucous membrane involvement with dysphagia; retinitis with 'cotton-wool' exudates; muscle weakness and tenderness including the posterior pharyngeal muscles; and acute pulmonary manifestations.

Differential diagnosis is mainly between polymyositis, dermatomyositis and a muscular dystrophy. The main difference is the absence of a rash in polymyositis and the usual lack of vasculitis. Muscular dystrophy may present a similar picture with symmetrical proximal muscle weakness. However, the muscles should not be tender and in the commonest type — pseudohypertrophic (Duchenne) muscular dystrophy — the muscles may show increased bulk. Rate of progress of the disease is generally slower in muscular dystrophy than dermatomyositis which may start acutely, but 50 per cent present with an insiduous form. Varying degrees of myositis occurs in other connective tissue disorders like rheumatoid arthritis, scleroderma and mixed connective tissue syndrome. These diagnoses should be considered. Investigation with EMG and muscle biopsy will discern between dermatomyositis/polymyositis and a muscular dystrophy. Autoantibodies, in particular anti-nuclear factor, may help to diagnose a connective tissue syndrome.

In the absence of a rash other disorders such as viral infections (in particular entero- and andenoviruses) toxoplasmosis and trichinosis must be entertained. Trichinosis is usually accompanied by an eosinophilia early in the disease. Bone marrow aspiration should always be done in a known leukaemic patient who presents with aches and pains in the limbs.

Further reading

Ansell, B. M. (ed.) (1980). The rarer connective tissue disorders. In *Rheumatic Disorders of Childhood*, p. 177. (London; Butterworths).
Devere, R. and Bradley, W. G. (1975). Polymyositis: its presentation, morbidity and mortality *Brain*, **98**, 637–666.
Sewell, J. R. (1982). Polymyositis and dermatomyositis. *Reports on Rheumatic Diseases*, January

Case 52

Answers

1. (a) Astrocytoma.
   (b) Medulloblastoma.

2. (a) Radioisotope scan.
   (b) CT scan.

Discussion

This girl has signs of raised intracranial pressure: headache with vomiting, papilloedema, raised blood pressure and erosion of the posterior clinoid process on skull X-ray. There are innumerable causes of raised intracranial pressure, but examination revealed a truncal ataxia, which suggests a lesion in the vermis of the cerebellum. The unsteady gait is also a feature of cerebellar space-occupying lesions. The most likely lesion is a tumour, either an astrocytoma or a medulloblastoma. Hydrocephalus producing raised intracranial pressure is produced early as the aqueduct is compromised, so signs of raised intracranial pressure may occur before localizing signs.

Medulloblastomas have a peak incidence between 1 and 5 years, are rapid growing and, therefore, present after a short history.

Astrocytomas have a peak incidence between 5 and 10 years, are are slow growing and present after a longer history. This is, therefore, the most likely diagnosis in this child.

Astrocytomas are usually benign lesions causing symptoms by slow growth, often with cyst formation. They may arise in the cerebellum, brain stem, third ventricle or cerebrum; the cerebellum is the commonest site.

The presenting signs of a cerebellar lesion are usually those of raised intracranial pressure with cerebellar signs developing subsequently. The history may be punctuated by periods of remission or conversely by rapid deterioration caused by a sudden increase in intracranial pressure by cysts blocking the ventricular system.

Brain-stem astrocytomas tend to be more diffuse so surgery is only indicated for decompression and radiotherapy is the treatment of choice. There is a classic triad of symptoms comprising multiple cranial nerve lesions, ataxia and pyramidal abnormalities. Signs of raised intracranial pressure tend to occur late.

Third-ventricle astrocytomas may present with hypothalamic dysfunction and visual loss from destruction of the surrounding structures and pressure on the optic chiasma. A lesion in the anterior wall of the third ventricle may produce the diencephalic syndrome of infancy. This syndrome often presents around 6 months of age with vomiting and extreme emaciation despite adequate calorie intake. Other features include sweating, hypoglycaemia, optic atrophy, nystagmus and a 'defiantly cheerful' demeanour.

Cerebral astrocytomas are rare in childhood and present with convulsions or signs of raised intracranial pressure after reaching a considerable size.

Medulloblastomas arise in the cerebellar vermis and expand rapidly into the fourth ventricle and cerebellar hemispheres causing cerebellar signs early in the history. Once the tumour is in the fourth ventricle, seeding may occur throughout the ventricular system. Seeding may also occur into the subarachnoid space producing a malignant meningitis and allowing the possibility of seeding in the spinal column causing such signs as back ache, lower limb weakness and bladder dysfunction. Distant metastases are rare and usually occur in the bone marrow. Treatment is by surgical excision and decompression of the hydrocephalus if necessary, followed by combined radiotherapy and chemotherapy.

Further reading

Gomez, M. A. and Reese, D. F. (1976). Computed tomography of the head in infants and children. *Pediatric Clinics of North America*, **23**, 473.

Merritt, H. H. (ed.) (1979). Tumours. In *A Textbook of Neurology*, 6th edn. p. 213. (Philadelphia; Lea and Febiger)

Richardon, A. (1979). Intracranial tumours. In *Paediatric Neurology*, Ed. by F. Clifford-Rose, p. 485. (Oxford; Blackwell Scientific Publications)

Walker, M. D. (1976). Diagnosis and treatment of brain tumours. *Pediatric Clinics of North America*, **23**, 131.

Case 53

Answers

1. (a) Lateral skull X-ray for intracerebral calcification.
   (b) Toxoplasma indirect fluorescent antibody titre.
   (c) Cytomegalovirus (CMV) specific IgM.
2. (a) Congenital *Toxoplasma gondii* infection.
   (b) Congenital CMV infection.
   (c) Congenital herpes hominis infection.

Discussion

The most likely cause of this child's neonatal problems is an intrauterine infection producing a week-long rash and prolonged jaundice. Microcephaly is commoner than hydrocephalus in congenital rubella, so the most likely infecting agents are CMV and toxoplasmosis. These would also explain the choroidoretinitis. A lateral skull X-ray may demonstrate intracerebral calcification. Classically this should be periventricular in CMV and diffuse in toxoplasmosis. Rarely disseminated congenital Herpes hominis infection causes intracranial calcification.

Toxoplasma gondii is a ubiquitous obligate intracellular parasite. The mode of spread is unclear; certainly this protozoon is rampant both in wild and in domestic animals. Uncooked meats may, therefore, be a source. The only animal found to pass infected faeces is the cat. Once infection occurs many organs are affected, which explains the diversity of the disease manifestations.

The congenitally acquired infection, transmitted transplacentally, may cause widespread cellular damage. The commonest sign is chroidoretinitis, which affects both macular and peripheral areas. Other features include convulsions, intracranial calcification hydrocephalus, anaemia, a petechial or maculopapular rash, prolonged neonatal jaundice, hepatosplenomegaly and an abnormal CSF. The CSF may be xanthochromic and display a leucocytosis, predominantly mononuclear; the protein may be raised to levels of up to 20 g. ℓ^{-1}.

The neurological damage is usually the most devastating although the organism is disseminated throughout the body. Meningoencephalomyelitis occurs, with large inflammatory lesions containing necrotic centres.

Eventually calcification and cyst formation occur. Areas involved are the cortex, subcortical white matter, caudate and lenticulate nuclei, mid-brain, pons, medulla oblongata and spinal cord. Hydrocephalus is caused by obstruction of the foramina of Munro or the aqueduct of Sylvius.

Fetal infection may cause a severe, rapidly fatal infection; however, less than 40 per cent of infants born to infected mothers are themselves infected, and of those only 11 per cent have overt disease.

Initially the toxoplasma dye test is positive and there is an increase in the indirect fluorescent antibody titre (IFA). Complement-fixing antibodies are absent initially but later rise to high levels. Maternal antibodies may cross the placenta and cause a high antibody titre in an uninfected infant. The titre will gradually fall over the first 4 months of life; in the infected infant the titre rises. The toxoplasma IFA titre will be raised in this child.

CMV, A DNA virus, is also widespread. Neonatal infection may be transplacental or via contact with infected cervical secretions. Only the minority of infants born to infected mothers have overt disease which may range from mild and self-limiting to fatal.

A diffuse petechial rash may occur within a few hours or days post-natally, secondary to thrombocytopenia, which usually clears rapidly but the hepatitis-induced jaundice may persist for up to 4 months. Neurological abnormalities include choroidoretinitis, spasticity, convulsions, microcephaly, hydrocephalus and cerebral calcification, usually periventricular. However, all major systems are involved causing cardiac, gastrointestinal and musculoskeletal abnormalities.

'Owl eye' cells, caused by intranuclear inclusion bodies, may be seen in the urine or the virus may be cultured in tissue culture. Immunological markers are the neutralizing antibody, indirect fluorescent antibody or complement fixation tests. The most rapid neonatal test is the detection of a raised CMV IgM titre, which is positive for several years.

Further reading

Krugman, S. and Katz, S. L. (eds) (1982). Toxoplasmosis. *Infectious Diseases of Children*, p. 417. (London; C. V. Mosby)

Krugman, S. and Katz, S. L. (eds) (1982). Cytomegalovirus infection. In *Infectious Diseases of Childhood*, p. 1. (London; C. V. Mosby)

Case 54

Answers

1. (a) The family history of migraine.
   (b) Associated symptoms of attacks, i. e. visual, headache, giddiness, motor, sensory, seizures and autonomic symptoms.
2. (a) EEG.
   (b) Therapeutic trial of ergotamine, propranolol or clonidine.

Discussion

The diagnosis here is migraine, but of a variant type. Differentiation from temporal lobe epilepsy can sometimes be difficult. All types of migraine occur in children: classic or common, in which an aura does not precede the headache; cluster headaches; hemiplegic; ophthalmoplegic and basilar artery migraine. Children with migraine equivalents may pose difficult problems in diagnosis. The most common is the recurrent abdominal syndrome in which there is recurrent abdominal pain with or without nausea, vomiting, cyclic vomiting, fever, chest pain, leg cramps and autonomic symptoms such as sweating, pallor, nasal congestion and eye watering. Headache, giddiness, photophobia and a confusional state with the child 'not quite himself' may also be present, but a good history can be notoriously difficult to obtain from a young child and his parents. A family history of migraine is present in a majority of children presenting with migraine. Pointers to this child having migraine are the sudden cessation of pain and vomiting after comparatively long episodes lasting 24 hours and lack of any type of seizures. Of course seizures do not always occur in temporal lobe epilepsy and may occur, usually focally, in migraine due to severe vasoconstriction. EEG abnormalities occur in about 20 per cent of patients with recurrent abdominal syndrome, so this investigation can be helpful to differentiate between migraine and epilepsy but if positive can be difficult to interpret. There is a sizeable amount of literature on the various abnormalities found in the EEG of migrainous patients.

There are no definite diagnostic procedures available, but a therapeutic trial of ergotamine may be tried early in the course of an attack. Propranolol can be used prophylactically in migraine and is effective in a number of children. Clonidine is also effective, but generally not recommended for children of this age by the manufacturers. Anticonvulsants may reduce the number of migraine attacks as well as epileptic episodes.

Antidepressants have at times been used with some effect in migraine since the number of attacks increases with depression. This was thought to be a factor in this child by his GP because of the decrease in attention from his mother due to illness in the fostered boy. This turned out not to be the case.

Porphyria should be considered in the differential diagnosis of abdominal pain in a child even though it is rare. The family history, possible precipitating factors and associated symptoms should be sought. Presentation with abdominal pain, vomiting, neuropsychiatric symptoms and finally muscular weakness or paralysis can make it very similar to migraine initially. Visual disturbances and convulsions occur late. On examination there is often marked tachycardia, hypertension and neurological abnormalities. In this case the diagnosis is unlikely in view of the normal urinary porphobilinogen result, although there are some very rare forms of porphyria in which this is raised only during an attack.

Further reading

Clifford-Rose, F. (ed.) (1979). *Paediatric Neurology*, 1st ed. pp. 373–386. (Oxford; Blackwell Scientific Publications)
Premsky, A. L. (1976). Migraine and migrainous variants in paediatric patients. *Pediatric Clinics of North America*, **23**, 373–380.
Burke, E. C. and Peters, G. A. (1956). Migraine in childhood. *American Journal of Diseases of Children*, **92**, 330–336.
Editorial (1980). Recurrent abdominal pain in childhood. *British Medical Journal*, **i**, 1096.
Beattie, A. and Goldberg, A. (1975). The porphyrias. *Medicine*, Series 1, **12**, 774–782.

Case 55

Answers

1. (a) Chest X-ray.
   (b) Sweat electrolytes.
   (c) Stool tryptic activity.
   (d) Repeated sputum culture.
   (e) Bronchography.
2. (a) Vigorous antibiotic therapy for each infection.
   (b) Physiotherapy.
   (c) Postural drainage.
   (d) Surgical excision.

Discussion

This child has chronic suppurative lung disease. He has a persistent purulent cough with haemoptysis, clubbing, ECG changes, and failure to thrive. The chest X-ray would show diffuse changes with bronchial widening and thickening consistent with bronchiectasis.

The commonest cause of this syndrome is cystic fibrosis. His stools were reported as normal, but as the only child he has no forerunners for comparison. Cystic fibrosis must, therefore, be excluded. Sweat electrolytes are diagnostic. Stool tryptic activity may be meausured but is normal in 10 per cent of cystics. His two earlier illnesses could be factors in the production of bronchiectasis. Pertussis, particularly, is associated with right middle-lobe collapse, often complicated by secondary bacterial invasion. Destructive changes occur rapidly in the bronchioles, producing bronchiectasis. If, however, the infection is treated promptly and the lobe re-expanded, the bronchiectatic changes resolve. Clinically, the presentation is similar to the above case except the crepitations should be localized.

An attack of bronchiolitis, especially if complicated by secondary bacterial infection, may produce slow progressive destruction of the bronchioles. Diffuse bronchiolar and parenchymal damage is caused, symptoms arise insidiously and crepitations would be heard at both bases.

Treatment is both prophylactic — with regular physio therapy, postural drainage and controlled coughing — and active, with prompt aggressive antibiotic therapy of exacerbations.

Surgery is only indicated once the disease process has stabilized, if the bronchiectasis is localized and if the child's symptoms are marked. It is difficult to determine the extent of bronchiectasis even on bronchography. Bronchiectatic changes have been demonstrated in bronchioles that were radiographically normal. Surgery must, therefore, be undertaken with care.

Further reading

Krugman, S. and Katz, S. L. (eds) (1982). Pertussis (whooping cough). In *Infectious Diseases of Children*, 7th edn. p. 246. (St Louis; Mosby)

Williams, H. E. and Phelan, P.D. (eds) (1975). Suppurative lung disease. In *Respiratory Disease in Children*, p. 197. (Oxford; Blackwell Scientific Publications)

Case 56

Answers

1. (a) Wilson's disease.
   (b) Chronic active hepatitis.

(c) Halothane hepatitis.
   (d) Non-A, non-B hepatitis.
   (e) α_1-Antitrypsin deficiency.
   (f) Other toxic injury — drugs, chemicals, plants.
2. (a) Serum caeruloplasmin.
   (b) Urinary copper excretion before and after penicillamine.
   (c) Slit lamp examintion for Kayser–Fleischer rings.
   (d) Protein electrophoretic strip.
   (e) α_1-Antitrypsin protease inhibitor phenotype.
   (f) Liver scan.
   (g) Halothane antibodies.
   (h) LE cells.
   (i) HLA type.
3. (a) Vitamin K.
   (b) Fresh frozen plasma.
   (c) Gut antibiotics, i.e. neomycin.
   (d) Lactulose.
   (e) Low-protein diet and vitamin supplementation.
   (f) Cimetidine.

Discussion

The possible diagnoses in this child range over a wide spectrum. The first impression is of an acute hepatitis with a high IgM at first, then rising IgG, but both HBS Ag and HAV IgM were negative. Non-A, non-B hepatitis is a possibilty, but no blood transfusion had been given to this boy, and this is thought to be the method of transmission. There may well be many viruses which are lumped together under the guise of 'non-A, non-B', with various modes of transmission; as yet there are no serological tests for diagnosis.

Halothane hepatitis is very uncommon in young children; out of 251 fully documented cases, only one was a child under 10 years. Usually multiple anaesthetics have been given and, generally, the last two within 28 days of each other. This was not so in this child, but he did develop vomiting and abdominal pain without jaundice after his previous anaesthetics. There is a test for halothane hepatitis where the serum of the patient is cytotoxic to halothane-treated rabbit hepatocytes. This is by no means foolproof. Halothane hepatitis is also associated with fever, eosinophilia and autoantibodies.

Several factors about this child should make one consider a chronic process. These are the markedly abnormal clotting tests, the dropping albumin level, the continually rising bilirubin value and high alkaline phosphatase activity despite dropping transaminase value, normal size but non-tender liver, and finally the length of history with episodes of vomiting, abdominal pain and 'abnormal' behaviour. Blood ammonia level would demonstrate the severity of liver damage and possible encephalopathy, while a liver scan would show the size of the liver plus normal or low uptake indicating a chronic reparative or acute necrosis, respectively. Wilson's disease and chronic active hepatitis are the most likely. Wilson's disease may present in childhood either as a chronic problem with cirrhosis, or acutely, such as in this case. It is very important to exclude it with caeruloplasmin and urinary copper estimations, also slit lamp examination. Neurological signs generally occur in the teens.

Chronic active hepatitis is rare before 6 years of age, approximately 70 per cent of cases are females and 60 per cent have HLA B8 tissue type. There are two types: HBS Ag positive and HBS Ag negative. The latter is a possibility here since it is associated with autoantibodies, in particular anti-nuclear factor (ANF), antimitochondrial, anti-thyroid, anti-liver-kidney microsomal and a high titre of smooth-muscle antibodies. Secondly, there are high titres of gammaglobulin, especially IgG. LE cells are present in 15 per cent of these patients.

α_1-Antitrypsin deficiency is a rare cause of childhood cirrhosis, but is unlikely here since very few patients develop significant liver disease without a history of obstructive jaundice in the first months of life. The easiest way to screen is with a protein electrophoretic strip, where a small band can be seen. The actual level may be measured, but diagnosis is made by finding which protease inhibitor (Pi) phenotype is present. PiZZ is the phenotype of α_1-Antitrypsin deficiency.

Treatment is aimed at correcting the clotting defects and reducing the possibility of hepatic encephalopathy by diet, gut decontamination and cimetidine to prevent bleeding.

Further reading

Inman, W. H. W. and Inman, W. W. (1978). Jaundice after repeated exposure to halothane — reports to the CSM. *British Medical Journal*, **ii**, 1455–1456.
Mowat, A. P. (1979). Childhood liver disease. *Medicine*, Series 3, **18**, 916.
Mowat, A. P. (1979). *Liver Disease in Childhood*, pp. 53–89, 94–109, 151–159, 215–232, 233–245. (London; Butterworths)
Vergani, D. *et al.* (1980). Antibodies to the surface of halothane-altered rabbit hepatocytes. *New England Journal of Medicine*, **303**, 66–71.
Zickerman, A. J. (1979). Viral hepatitis. *Medicine*, Series 3, **18**, 903.

Case 57

Answers

1. Enlarged adenoids and tonsils sufficient to cause hypercapnoea with subsequent pulmonary vasoconstriction and hypertension.

Discussion

This child has clinical and cardiographic evidence of right ventricular hypertrophy with pulmonary hypertension and increased right ventricular pressures on catheter studies. There is no evidence of a left-to-right shunt and the right atrial pressure is only minimally raised; this suggests a pulmonary vascular cause of the hypertension. The child was a mouth-breather (indicating large adenoids), the episodes occurred when the child relaxed whilst on her back, and upper respiratory tract infections exacerbated the problem. It is possible, therefore, that the airway was sufficiently embarrassed by hypertrophied adenoids and tonsils to cause chronic hypercapnoea and subsequent pulmonary vasoconstriction and hypertension. When the child relaxed the hypertrophied adnexa closed the airway completely. Continued hypertension and increased right-sided pressures result in ventricular hypertrophy; atrial hypertrophy will occur if the ventricular diastolic pressure rises. Vascular response includes an increase in the arterial muscle mass and distal muscular extension. These changes eventually become permanent with irreversible haemodynamic changes. However, diminution of the muscle mass and haemodynamic equilibrium are restored if the initiating cause is removed promptly, particularly before the age of 2 years.

Pulmonary hypertension also occurs in response to increased pulmonary blood flow as in a left-to-right shunt. Similar physical and haemodynamic consequences occur, again reversible initially. If uncorrected, right-sided pressures may equal and pass systemic pressures causing reversal of the shunt with cyanosis, the Eisenmenger's syndrome. Careful monitoring of such affected children is, therefore, mandatory.

Further reading

Jordan, S. C. and Scott, O. (eds) (1973). Pulmonary hypertension, cor pulmonale and the Eisenmenger's syndrome. In *Heart Disease in Paediatrics*, p. 220. (London; Butterworths)

Macartney, F. J. (1979). Heart and circulation. In *Clinical Paediatric Physiology*, p. 304. (Oxford; Blackwell Scientific Publications)

Case 58

Answers

1. Limb-girdle muscular dystrophy.
2. (a) Creatinine phosphokinase (CPK) activity.
   (b) EMG.
   (c) Muscle biopsy.

Discussion

The main differential diagnosis in this case is between limb-girdle muscular dystrophy and chronic polymyositis. Myopathies frequently present with weakness of the girdle musculature. Early difficulties include lifting, carrying, throwing, combing the hair, running, getting up from a squatting position off the floor or a low chair and climbing stairs. Walking is often unimpaired but patients may have a waddling gait and experience sudden falls due to weakness of the quadriceps. The pattern of muscle wasting is of diagnostic importance; selective atrophy of individual muscles suggests muscular dystrophy while more diffuse wasting and weakness suggests an acquired myopathy or one of the more benign congenital myopathies such as central core disease. The history above is non-specific, pain may occur in myopathic muscles especially if they are hypertrophied initially. Pain can occur in limb-girdle dystrophy which is inherited as an autosomal recessive but is more common in Duchenne's muscular dystrophy which is sex linked. The pain is more marked on exercise and weakness may well be increased at the end of the day. Limb-girdle dystrophy occurs generally in two forms: the pelvifemoral or the scapulo humeral depending on which limb girdle is primarily affected. On examination, however, there are usually clinical signs of wasting and weakness in both girdles as in the patient described. Diagnosis is aided by the investigations outlined. The CPK is moderately elevated and muscle biopsy shows non-specific dystrophic changes. EMG should show a myopathic picture.

Chronic polymyositis begins insidiously, with increasing weakness over weeks, months or years. In contrast to muscular dystrophy, weakness is more diffuse, wasting less pronounced, tendon reflexes preserved and muscle tenderness more common. Other features may be transient rashes, flitting arthralgias and

Raynaud's phenomenon. Polymyositis alone, without skin involvement, is relatively uncommon in childhood. CPK is raised in approximately 70 per cent of patients, an EMG will indicate myopathy with fibrillation potentials and muscle biopsy shows fibres undergoing necrosis and phagocytosis with collections of inflammatory cells. ANF is often positive. Systemic lupus erythematosus is an outside possibility, but negative ANF and RF results make this unlikely.

Other diagnoses that should be considered in a possible limb-girdle dystrophy are: the benign form of spinal muscular atrophy of Kugelberg and Welander, which should present at an earlier age and is commonly associated with tremor of the hands; secondly, acid maltase deficiency (type II glycogenosis) which in childhood or adult form, not infantile (Pompe's disease), is very similar. However, the heart and respiratory muscles may be affected leading to respiratory insufficiency. Muscle biopsy is diagnostic.

Painful muscles at rest occur in other conditions in children. These include trichinosis which causes muscle pain, weakness and general malaise associated with as eosinophilia; acute myoglobinuric myopathies and myopathies of metabolic bone disease. The former is usually episodic and acute, related to exercise, infection or toxin, while the latter causes only minimal wasting with normal or hyperactive tendon reflexes. CPK, EMG and serum calcium may all be normal, but alkaline phosphatase activity is invariably raised.

Further reading

Ansell, B. M. (ed.) (1980). The rarer connective tissue disorders. In *Rheumatic disorders in Childhood*, pp. 167–212. (London; Butterworths)
Dubowitz, V. (ed.) (1978). Muscle disorders in childhood. In *Major Problems in Clinical Pediatrics*, Vol. **XVI**, Chaps. 1–4. (Philadelphia; Saunders)
Morgan-Hughes, J. (1980). Diseases of muscle. *Medicine*, Series 3, **34**, 1719–1731.

Case 59

Answers

1. Digoxin level.
2. Plasma potassium.

Discussion

Digoxin has several effects on the depolarization wave in cardiac muscle. Phase 4, depolarization, has an increased slope, decreasing the time of depolarization and increasing the automaticity of the fibres. This effect of digoxin is a function of intracellular potassium, increased automaticity and excitability of cardiac fibres, eventually causing ectopic beats. In this child the extracellular potassium level was markedly reduced by the diuretic action of theophylline whereas the digoxin level of 1.5 ng. ml^{-1} was normal. This combination led to coupled beats. The xanthines, theophylline and 1, 3, dimethylxanthine, probably cause a diuresis by inhibiting the reabsorption of sodium and chloride in the proximal convoluted tubule. This allows greater sodium/potassium exchange in the distal convoluted tubule.

The cellular basis of action of the xanthines has not been fully elucidated. Three possible actions have been suggested. The first relates to the translocation of intracellular calcium. This may account for the stimulation of cardiac and striated muscle. However, smooth muscle, especially bronchial muscle, is relaxed. Secondly, the xanthines inhibit phosphodiesterase, increasing intracellular cyclic AMP; this may account for excitation of the central nervous system producing decreased tiredness and more efficient functioning. The third mechanism is the block of adenosine receptors. Adenosine may act via cyclic AMP or be totally independent of it. The effects of adenosine include dilatation of the blood vessels, especially coronary and cerebral, and slowing of the rate of discharge of the cardiac pacemaker cells and some neurones in the central nervous system. However, the clincial effects of theophylline include constriction of the cerebral vasculature and stimulation of cardiac fibres and the central nervous system. There must obviously be complex cellular interactions before the clinical effects of theophylline are manifest.

Further reading

Hoffman, B. F. and Bigger, J. T. (1975). Cardiovascular drugs. In *The Pharmacological Basis of Therapeutics*, Ed. by A. Gilman and L. S. Goodman, 6th edn., p. 732. (New York; MacMillan Publishing)

Murphy, J. E. (1979). The current role of oral theophylline derivatives in respiratory medicine. *Journal of International Medical Research*, **7**, Supplement 1.

Rall, T. W. (1975). The xanthines. In *The Pharmacological Basis of Therapeutics*, Ed. by A. Gilman and L. S. Goodman, 6th edn., p. 596. (New York; MacMillan Publishing)

Case 60

Answers

1. (a) Skull X-rays.
    (b) CT scan.
    (c) Visual fields.
    (d) Serum T_3 and T_4.
2. (a) Hypothalamic tumour (diencephalic syndrome of childhood)
    (b) Psychosocial deprivation.
3. (a) Shunt procedure for hydrocephalus.
    (b) Radiotherapy.

Discussion

Many causes of failure to thrive have been eliminated in this child: i.e. cystic fibrosis, heart disease, coeliac disease or malabsorption syndrome (very unlikely in view of the normal xylose absorption test). Chronic infection is a possibility but the apparent well-being of the child is against this. The differential diagnosis lies between psychosocial deprivation and an intracranial lesion. There are certainly sufficient factors in the family and social history to fit with emotional deprivation, but this child always appeared very happy and on admission to hospital did not gain weight as expected with a change of environment and regular feeding. His height on the 25th centile and weight on the 3rd is also against this diagnosis. One would expect short stature in keeping with the weight.

An intracranial lesion is therefore the most likely diagnosis. In view of the history and absence of neurological signs apart from congenital nystagmus, a hypothalamic tumour is most likely. When the tumour is in the anterior wall of the 3rd ventricle the infants are either anorexic or have a voracious appetite and become progressively emaciated while remaining bright, happy and active. Hydrocephalus may be symptomless, skin depigmentation is usual, hypotension and hypoglycaemia may occur; growth hormone levels have been reported as grossly elevated. With tumours of other areas of the hypothalamus the optic chiasma and nerves are encroached on early. This results in visual-field defects and optic atrophy. In this case the nystagmus may have been due to disturbed macular vision secondary to the tumour but optic atrophy was not noted. Hydrocephalus is progressive as a result of 3rd ventricle invasion and requires treatment. The tumour is an astrocytoma and since it is inaccessible to surgery, treatment is with radiotherapy.

Useful investigations are limited. Skull X-rays may show separation of the sutures; visual fields would be extremely difficult if not impossible in such a child; but a CT scan is mandatory. If this is not available, investigations such as isotope brain scan and pneumoencephalography can be done.

Hyperthyroidism is a possibility, but in this age group very rare, especially with no goitre or eye signs. It is most common in adolescent females who develop thyroid antibodies. Serum levels of T_3 and T_4 are usually elevated.

Further reading

Bailey, J. D., Ehrleich, R. M., Fraser, D. and Howard, A. (1978). *Medicine, Series 2*, No 10, Short Stature, 465; Thyroid Function during childhood, p. 480.
Clifford-Rose, F. (ed.) (1979). *Paediatric Neurology*, 1st edn., p. 437. (London; Butterworths)
Torrey, E. F. (1965). Diencephalic syndrome of infancy. American Journal of Diseases in Childhood, **110**, 689.

Case 61

Answers

1. (a) Typhoid.
    (b) Paratyphoid.
2. (a) Blood culture.
    (b) Widal's agglutination test.
    (c) Stool culture.
    (d) Urine culture.
3. (a) Chloramphenicol.
    (b) Co-trimoxazole.
    (c) Amoxycillin.

Discussion

Typhoid in children can present in a number of unusual ways, often just as a pyrexia of unknown origin (PUO) with no accompanying diarrhoea. This child presents a fairly typical picture of early typhoid with abdominal pain, fever, headache and cough. The signs on examination are generally non-specific. Meningism is sometimes present, together with mental confusion, but examination of the CSF is usually normal. It is well recognized that there can be positive findings on clinical examination of the chest, but the chest X-ray is often surprisingly clear. Leucopenia is common in typhoid, although it is also present in a viral infection or overwhelming bacterial infection.

Jaundice can be one of the initial presentations of typhoid fever due to haemolysis and anaemia is common. Raised transaminase activities are often non-specific findings.

As the illness proceeds, the temperature rises. Although convulsions are not very common they do occur, especially in children. More common complications are gastrointestinal haemorrhage and perforation.

Paratyphoid fever can present with a similar picture to typhoid fever but is usually less severe. Lassa fever, only found in Nigeria, also presents with a similar course.

Other diagnoses that may be considered are shigella dysentery which generally presents with diarrhoea and possibly dehydration, but a young child may be toxic and have meningism. Blood in the stool with abdominal pain occurs with giardiasis, campylobacter, and amoebiasis, but the children are not markedly pyrexial and meningism does not occur. Yersinia enterocolitis gives a clinical picture varying from mesenteric adenitis to acute diarrhoea of brief duration.

Salmonella typhi should be grown from a blood culture. It can also be isolated from the stools and urine but this does not prove the diagnosis unequivocally since the patient may be a carrier with an unrelated illness, although this coincidence is unusual. A rising titre on Widal's agglutination test in a patient who has not received TAB vaccine recently is good evidence in favour of typhoid fever.

Chloramphenicol is still the mainstay of treatment despite the complication of marrow aplasia. Co-trimoxazole has been used fairly extensively for fully sensitive organisms and is usually free from marrow toxicity. Amoxycillin is also effective and may be important in the treatment of the chronic carrier state.

Further reading

British Medical Journal (1979). Typhoid fever. British Medical Journal, **i**, 213.
Mandal, B. K. (1981). Intestinal infections in adults and children over the age of two. *Medicine*, Series 4, **2**, 56.
Nye, F. J. and Bell, D. R. (1978). Gastro-intestinal infections. *Medicine*, Series 3, **5**, 234.
Ramsay, A. M. and Emond, R. T.D. (1967). *Infectious Diseases*, pp. 189–202. (London, Heinemann).

Case 62

Answers

1. Poliomyelitis.
2. (a) Stool and pharyngeal washings for viruses.
   (b) Serum antibody titres for polioviruses.
3. (a) Bed rest for child during acute phase.
   (b) Report case to District Medical Officer.
   (c) Make sure that encampment is fully immunized (this should be done by Public Health Inspector).
   (d) Watch for respiratory and bulbar complications.
   (e) Physiotherapy in recovery phase.

Discussion

Other diagnoses which should be considered here besides poliomyelitis are Guillain–Barré syndrome (GBS), peripheral neuropathy and acute encephalopathy. In GBS there is often a preceding viral illness but the paralysis usually progresses slowly over 1–2 weeks, while in polio paralysis progresses quickly; the final extent can usually be asssessed in 48–72 hours. Secondly, in GBS there is symmetrical paralysis, usually sensory symptoms, a high CSF protein and low cell count, while in polio paralysis is classically asymmetrical and there are no sensory symptoms. CSF protein is normal and cell count consistent with viral meningitis. Both conditions have muscle pain preceding paralysis; this can vary considerably in its severity but is usually more marked in GBS.

Peripheral neuropathy of acute onset may also be due to: porphyria (which is most unlikely in a child so young), diphtheria (in which aseptic meningitis does not develop and which generally causes severe constitutional upset), toxins such as lead and other heavy metals or drugs such as isoniazid (these should always be kept in mind when dealing with a poorly supervised child), serum sickness after immunization and malignancy.

Encephalopathy is usually secondary to infection, either bacterial or viral. Blood count here is more in favour of a viral infection; of particular note are EB virus, CMV, herpes simplex, ECHO virus and arboviruses. Asphyxia, haemorrhage, toxins and metabolic disease also cause an encephalopathy, but generally presentation is with fits, coma and hemiplegia.

Diagnosis is by isolation of the virus. Stools are the best material, although throat washings are of use in the first week. It is rarely isolated from the CSF and a lumbar puncture should not be attempted once the paralytic stage has been reached since paralysis is more common at sites of recent trauma; for example bulbar palsy is more likely after tonsillectomy. There is a fourfold rise in antibody titre to the isolated virus in acute and convalescent serum.

In a sporadic case such as this, reporting of the case to Public Health Authorities is of primary importance. This could be either a wild virus or an attenuated virus from another child who has recently been immunized. It is important that the gypsy camp population is screened and immunized, since this will stop the spread of the virus. For the child, nursing care in the acute phase consists of keeping the full range of movement in the limbs, prevention of bed sores and of chest infection, respiratory and bulbar paralysis. Once the acute phase of increasing paralysis has passed active physiotherapy to try to regain as much movement as possible should be given.

Further reading

Brown, K. (1980). Acute encephalopathies of childhood. *Medicine*, Series 3, **33**, 1702.
Christie, A. B. (1981). Poliomyelitis. *Medicine*, Series 4, **4**, 138.
McLeod, J. G. (1980). Peripheral neuropathy. *Medicine*, Series 3, **34**, 1755.
Ramsay, A. M. and Emond, R. T. D. (1967). Poliomyelitis. In *Infectious Diseases*, pp. 120–132. (London, Heinemann).

Case 63

Answers

1. Hyponatraemia.
2. (a) Serum sodium level.
   (b) Serum osmolality

Discussion

The mother had received a large volume of hypotonic fluid for her size and, in addition, had had an oxytocin infusion. Oxytocin has a slight intrinsic antidiuretic action, causing expansion of the maternal and, therefore, the fetal extracellular fluid compartments. The term newborn infant has a low renal blood flow and glomerular filtration rate, even when corrected for surface area. This reduces the ability of the kidney to excrete a water load. The child was born at approximately 36 weeks' gestation. However, his birth weight was 3rd centile for 36 weeks but at the 50th centile for 32 weeks' gestation. This prematurity would effect a concomitant reduction in renal maturity. The serum sodium in this child was 116 mmol. ℓ^{-1}. Serum osmolality would be low but would not indicate which of the osmotically active agents was so deficient. The treatment is to correct the serum sodium concentration with hypertonic sodium infusion over 6–10 hours.

Maturation of the kidney is both anatomical and hormonal. Renal blood flow and glomerular filtration rate increase rapidly. The neonatal loop of Henle is shorter than the adult, permitting a maximal urinary concentration of 50–60 per cent of the adult, despite the slow fluid flow facilitating solute reabsorption. Growth of the loop of Henle is rapid in the first 9 months of life.

The distal convuluted tubule and collecting ducts are relatively insensible to anti-diuretic hormone (ADH). ADH acts via cyclic AMP, which rises only modestly in the neonate. Again maturation occurs rapidly in the first few months of life. The immature kidney, therefore, is inefficient at excreting either a high solute load or high water load.

Further reading

Chantler, C. (1979). The Kidney In *Clinical Paediatric Physiology*, Ed. by S. Godfrey and J. D. Baum, p. 366. (Oxford, Blackwell Scientific Publications).

Oh, W. (1976). Disorders of fluid and electrolytes in newborn infants. *Paediatric Clinics of North America*, **23**, 601.
Spitzer, A. (1978). Renal physiology and functional development. In *Paediatric Kidney Disease*, Ed. by C. M. Edelman, p. 89. (Boston; Little, Brown).

Case 64

Answers

1. Immunoglobulins.
2. (a) Broad-spectrum antibiotics in combination such as amino-glycoside + carbenicillin/cephalosporin, taking into account any cultures and sensitivities known.
   (b) Correct fluid and electrolytes balance, then consider nutrition with either an elemental diet or parenteral feeding.
   (c) Irradiated blood transfusion.
   (d) Irradiated buffy coat transfusion.
   (e) Gamma globulin.
3. Severe combined immune deficiency.

Discussion

The relevant points in this patient's history are the recurrent infections and failure to thrive, with gastrointestinal symptoms in the presence of lymphopenia. Any child, especially a boy, who has recurrent infection should have their immunoglobulins investigated since hypogammaglobulinaemia is x-linked. In contrast to infants with severe combined immune deficiency (SCID), boys with hypogammaglobulinaemia have lymph nodes, tonsils and adenoids, a thymus on chest X-ray, but no lymphopenia. B- and T-lymphocyte markers will show lack of surface immunoglobulins on B cells but normal numbers of E rosettes, indicating the presence of T cells. T-cell function is intact. Other x-linked conditions are chronic granulomatous disease which generally presents with recurrent skin infections, osteomyelitis and hepatosplenomegaly; Wiskott–Aldrich syndrome presenting with infections, thrombocytopenia and eczema, and SCID which can also be inherited as an autosomal recessive.

Gastrointestinal symptoms are common in immune-deficient states. Combined IgG, IgA and IgM deficiencies (x-linked hypogammaglobulinaemia) cause symptoms in 14–50 per cent of cases, according to different series, but these disorders are usually minor. Thymic dysplasia and diminished cellular immunity may be associated with severe diarrhoea, disaccharidase deficiency, bacterial overgrowth, *Giardia lambli* infestations and malnutrition. A child with SCID may thus be expected to have severe gastrointestinal symptoms with refractory failure to thrive. Other presentations include recurrent respiratory infections, including *Pneumocystis carinii*, candidal infections of skin, mouth and gut, chronic otitis media and recurrent skin infections. Clinically there is no lymphoid tissue including thymus, no hepatosplenomegaly, and an absolute lymphopenia of both B and T cells with low or absent immunoglobulins and defective T-cell function. If blood products are given unirradiated, a graft-versus-host (GVH) reaction will occur.

Treatment of an immune-compromised patient follows general lines at first with eradication of infection as far as possible. Initially, broad-spectrum antibiotics, an aminoglycoside and pseudomonas-sensitive penicillin are used. In penicillin-sensitive patients a cephalosporin is used. Antibiotics are changed or added to, to take into account any positive cultures and sensitivities. Gut decontamination can be employed to reduce the carriage rate of possible pathogens. First, candida prophylaxis with amphotericin or miconazole, and secondly neomycin/Colomycin (colistin and colistin sulphomethrate) or co-trimoxazole for bacteria. In this case it is necessary to give prophylaxis for pneumocystis, thus co-trimoxazole is the treatment of choice.

Secondly, it is important to regain fluid and electrolyte balance followed by improved nutrition prior to carrying out a possible curative procedure such as bone marrow transplantation. Parenteral feeding would probably be necessary at first followed by an elemental diet designed to cater for any intolerances.

All blood products must be irradiated otherwise fatal GVH reactions may occur. Buffy coat can be very useful for eradicating an infection in conjunction with antibiotics. Gamma globulin may be useful.

Further reading

Amman, A. J., et al. (1975). Evaluation of infants and children with recurrent infection. *Current Problems in Pediatrics*, **5**, 3–47.
Anderson, C. M. and Barke, V. (1975). *Paediatric Gasto-enterology*, 1st ed. pp. 230–233, 571–595. (London: Blackwells)

Gelfard, E. W., et al. (1974). Immune deficiency: evaluation, diagnosis, and therapy. *Pediatric Clinics of North America*, **21**, 745–776.
Rosen, F. S. (1974). Primary immunodeficiency. *Pediatric Clinics of North America*, **21**, 533–549.

Case 65

Answers

1. Postnatal extrahepatic biliary atresia.
2. α_1-antitrypsin deficiency.

Discussion

This infant has evidence of a worsening cholestatic jaundice first noticed shortly after birth. Conjugated hyperbilirubinaemia has multiple causes including infection, inborn errors of metabolism and biliary atresia. No evidence of pre- or post-natal infection was detected; this, however, does not preclude a diagnosis of hepatitis as many cases have no cause determined. No evidence of galactosaemia or fructosaemia was found. Again this does not preclude these diagnoses as patients may not have galactosuria or fructosuria for several months. Obviously the patient must have ingested the relevant disaccharide.

Liver biopsy revealed proliferation of the bile ductules with an inflammatory exudate. This histology is compatible with extrahepatic biliary atresia and α_1-antitrypsin deficiency. Multinucleated giant cells are more commonly associated with hepatitis, but may be seen in both conditions. The infant was of normal birth weight, whereas the majority of patients with α_1-antitrypsin activity are of low birth weight.

Congenital biliary atresia produces a similar histological appearance, but is unlikely as this child was not jaundiced from birth. Postnatal biliary atresia is, therefore, more likely.

The incidence of extrahepatic biliary atresia is approximately 1 in 14 000 live births; the aetiology is unknown. It is postulated that the precipitating insult initiates a sclerosing inflammatory lesion in the ductular tissues. This may occur in fetal, perinatal or early postnatal life, allowing, as in this case, a picture of hepatitis superseded by that of atresia. 25 per cent of cases of extrahepatic biliary atresia have associated congenital malformations; however, no one system is implicated. Diagnosis should be made rapidly as results indicate that operative procedures should be performed before 80 days of age to carry a reasonable prognosis. Diagnosis should be made with a combination of clinical suspicion, a low excretion of [I^{131}] Rose Bengal dye and a characteristic biopsy. Ultrasound is only helpful in determining the presence of large extrahepatic masses and will not detect the absence of a biliary tree. Laparotomy may be necessary to determine a definitive diagnosis. The operation of choice is hepatic portoenterostomy, allowing bile to drain into a blind-ending loop of jejunum. There is no effective medical treatment and death usually supervenes within 2 years without surgery.

α_1-Antitrypsin deficiency is a rare disease causing hepatitis with subsequent cirrhosis and emphysema. α_1-Antitrypsin is an acute-phase protein, levels rise during infection, surgery or pregnancy. There are several phenotypes. PiM is the most common normal globulin. Those suffering from the disease commonly have either the phenotype PiZZ or Pi null, with no α_1-antitrypsin. Not all patients with deficiency suffer symptoms, and other genetic control factors have been postulated to explain these observations.

Initially the liver biopsy may resemble that of extrahepatic biliary atresia. However, after 12 weeks of age characteristic intracellular deposits are noted. Clinical presentation is varied, ranging from mild icterus with slow weight gain to marked failure to thrive, vomiting, hypotension and septicaemia. Survivors of the acute phase later develop cirrhosis. The onset of pulmonary symptoms usually occurs in the third or fourth decade; however, a few cases of childhood and adolescent onset have been reported. No effective treatment is available.

Further reading

Mowat, A. P. (ed.) (1979). Conjugated hyperbilirubinaemia. In *Liver Disorders in Childhood*, p. 53. (London; Butterworths)
Mowat, A. P. (ed.) (1979). Extrahepatic biliary atresia. In *Liver Disorders in Childhood*, p. 78. (London; Butterworths)
Williams, H. G. and Phelan, P. D. (eds) (1975). Uncommon lung diseases. II. In *Respiratory Illness in Children*, p. 349. (Oxford; Blackwell Scienfitic Publications)

Case 66

Answers

1. Glucose-6-phosphate dehydrogenase (G6PD) deficiency.
2. (a) G6PD level in RBCs.
   (b) Fluorescent spot test.
   (c) Haptoglobins.
   (d) Urine for Hb urobilinogen.
   (e) Coomb's test.
   (f) Chest X-ray.
   (g) Liver function tests.
3. (a) Sulphonamides.
   (b) Nitrofurantoin.
   (c) Fava beans.
   (d) Primaquine.
   (e) Naphthalene.

Discussion

This boy presents a picture of acute haemolysis with anaemia, reticulocytosis and jaundice. There are also features of intravascular haemolysis with fragmented RBCs and haemoglobulinuria (dark urine); urobilinogen is not dark. Bite cells occur in small numbers during oxidant haemolysis and have the same significance as Heinz bodies, being aggregates of oxidized and denatured Hb attached to the red cell membrane. The absence of spherocytes suggests that the haemolysis is not autoimmune, these being invariably found in warm antibody haemolytic anaemia. Any other diagnosis that might be considered such as hepatitis, nephritis or leukaemia does not fit the clinical picture, i.e. normal coloured stools, normal urea and electrolytes, low blood pressure and good marrow response to anaemia.

The most common cause of oxidant haemolysis is G6PD deficiency, especially in a boy of near-oriental or Mediterranean origin. It is inherited as a sex-linked recessive. Haemolysis may occur spontaneously but generally is secondary to drugs such as primaquine and sulphonamides. Fava beans, a staple dietary component of Mediterranean people, cause haemolysis, the condition being called 'favism'. This boy had been seen eating a small piece of mothball (naphthalene), also well recognized to cause haemolysis. Infections such as hepatitis or pneumonia may caus' haemolytic episodes in deficient individuals, hence the relevance of a chest X-ray and liver function tests.

Diagnosis is best made by measuring the level of G6PD in the red cells. However, a good screening test is a fluorescent spot test which is based on the reduction by haemolysate of nicotinamide adenine dinucleotide (NADP) to NADPH which fluoresces under ultraviolet light. G6PD-deficient red cells cannot produce the reduced NADPH and thus no fluorescent spot appears on the filter paper. Other investigations which are appropriate for any patient with haemolytic anaemia are: the Coombs' test which, if positive, means autoantibodies are present; haptoglobin level which should be reduced since it complexes with free Hb released by haemolysis, and urine for urobilinogen and Hb — if one suspects intravascular haemolysis. A positive Schumm test indicates elevation of plasma Hb and its oxidation product, methaemalbumin. No further information is gained by doing this test.

Other causes of intravascular haemolysis are paroxysmal nocturnal haemoglobinuria (PNH) and paroxysmal cold haemoglobinuria, both very unusual in this age group, and mechanical haemolysis from a prosthetic heart valve. The history does not suggest any of these diagnoses.

Further reading

De Gruchy, D. C. (1972). Haemolytic anaemia associated with glucose-6-phosphate dehydrogenase deficiency. In *Clinical Haematology in Medical Practice*, pp. 342–345. (London; Blackwell)

Sullivan, D. W. and Glader, B. E. (1980). Erythrocyte enzyme disorders in children. *Pediatric Clinics of North America*. **27**, 449–462.

Wiley, J. S. (1980). Haemolysis. *Medicine*, Series 3, **28**, 1468–1473.

Willoughby, M. L. N. (1977). Hereditary non-spherocytic haemolytic anaemias (enzyme deficiencies). In *Pediatric Haematology*, pp. 92–97. (Edinburgh; Churchill Livingstone)

Case 67

Answers

1. (a) Tracheo-oesophageal fistula.
   (b) Oesophageal stricture, e.g. vascular ring.

(c) Achalasia of the cardia.
    (d) Hiatus hernia.
    (e) Tracheo-oesophageal cleft.
    (f) Pharyngeal pouch.
2. (a) Cineradiography during barium swallow.
    (b) Bronchoscopy.

Discussion

Recurrent chest infections have a multiplicity of aetiologies. Such possibilities include a left-to-right shunt, lung parenchymal damage, immune deficiency and recurrent inhalation. Many aspects of this history suggest inhalation. Coughing occurred intermittently from birth, sometimes associated with feeding. Eventually the cough became persistent and wheezing was noted. Chest X-ray changes were restricted to both lower lobes which are the areas affected by inhalation while upright. Corroborative evidence included normal immunoglobulins, sweat test, stool trypsin activity and absence of a cardiovascular abnormality.

A common cause of inhalation is palatal and pharyngeal incoordination especially in the premature or in those with neurological damage. At 37 weeks' gestation, poor palatal control may occur. However, coordination should rapidly develop in the absence of neurological deficit, as in this child who is developmentally and neurologically normal. Inhalation may occur secondary to congenital abnormalities. Tracheo-oesophageal fistula permits the passage of foodstuffs to the lungs. A large fistula would cause catastrophic results which may be fatal; if the lumen is narrow only small amounts of fluid pass. As this continues the reflex coughing may diminish and it may be difficult to relate the episodes to feeding. A rare variation of abnormal foregut development is a tracheo-oesophageal cleft, where the two structures fail to separate. The cleft may be insignificant or extend to the pharynx or bronchi.

Stasis or interruption of the passage of food as in achalasia or stricture of the oesophagus facilitates inhalation. Regurgitation into the oropharynx permitted by a hiatus hernia, especially when recumbent, allows inhalation. Rarely a pharyngeal pouch may be implicated.

The association of coughing with feeding suggest the most likely diagnoses are a tracheo-oesophageal fistula and achalasia or stricture of the oesophagus.

Diagnosis of the 'H' tracheo-oesophageal fistula, which accounts for only 8 per cent of such abnormalities, may present severe problems. Cineradiography during a swallow may or may not outline the fistula transiently. Bronchoscopy, however, should reveal the abnormal opening. Rarely, fistulas may exist from the oesophagus or stomach to the bronchi.

The most common form of tracheo-oesophageal fistula is with a blind-ending proximal oesophageal pouch and a fistula from the trachea to the distal oesophagus. Diagnosis should be made rapidly as the infant can swallow nothing. Surgery is indicated in all these abnormalities. Unfortunately, even though anastomosis may be possible, oesophageal peristalsis is usually abnormal, with resulting repeated inhalation. Approximately 20 per cent of cases are associated with other congenital abnormalities, usually in the renal, cardiovascular or gastrointestinal systems.

Further reading

Cudmore, R. E. (1978). Oesophageal atresia and tracheo oesophageal fistula. In *Neonatal Surgery*, Ed. by P. P. Rickham, J. Lister and I. M. Irving, 2nd edn. p. 189. (London; Butterworths)
Lister, J. and Rickham, P. P. (1978). Hiatus hernia and chalasia of the cardia. In *Neonatal Surgery*, Ed. by P. P. Rickham, J. Lister and I. M. Irving, 2nd edn. p. 179. (London; Butterworths)
Williams, H. E. and Phelan, P. D. (1975). Pulmonary complications of inhalation. In *Respiratory Illness in Children*, p. 243. (Oxford; Blackwell Scientific Publications)

Case 68

Answers

1. (a) Reducing substances.
   (b) Red cell enzymes.
   (c) Insulin levels.
   (d) Urinary amino acids.
   (e) Toxoplasmosis, others, rubella, cytomegalovirus, herpes (TORCH) antibodies.
2. Von Gierke's disease (type I glycogenosis).

Discussion

Neonatal hypoglycaemia, usually defined as a blood glucose level of less than 1.6 mmol. ℓ^{-1} in the term infant, is a common problem. Several categories of infants are 'at risk' including the premature, small for gestational age and infants of diabetic mothers. Certain perinatal catastrophes such as intraventricular haemorrhages, rhesus incompatability and neonatal cold injury also predispose to hypoglycaemia. However, this infant is an apparently healthy full-term child who rapidly develops resistant hypoglycaemia, shortly after being fed. Although early, it is important to exclude galactosaemia.

The older sibling died in the early neonatal period, suggesting an inherited disorder, possibly of amino acid metabolism or metabolite storage. A mild metabolic acidosis was noted and also hepatosplenomegaly; these features would be explained by a glycogen storage disease, especially type I — von Gierke's disease.

The determination of insulin levels would be useful to differentiate failure of utilization, such as enzyme defects, from causes with excess insulin, such as β-cell adenomatosis and erythroblastosis fetalis.

Von Gierke's disease is caused by a deficiency of glucose-6-phosphatase which inhibits the release of glucose from glycogen or gluconeogenesis. The symptoms, therefore, relate to the subsequent hypoglycaemia. The infantile presentation is the least common but most severe variant. Control of the hypoglycaemia may be extremely difficult, occasionally requiring intravenous alimentation or a portocaval shunt. Even so, the mortality rate in the first year of life is high. Presentation may be via apnoeic episodes, vomiting or failure to thrive; convulsions may occur. Fatty infiltration of the liver is progressive and a bleeding diathesis with thrombocytosis may be a complicating factor.

Biochemical changes secondary to the hypoglycaemia include hyperlipidaemia from β lipolysis, ketosis and lactic acidosis and hyperuricaemia, probably due to a renal transport defect secondary to hyperlactataemia.

Increasing glycogen deposition causes progressive hepatosplenomegaly and bony changes with thinning of the cortex and widening of the medulla.

The combination of the above biochemical abnormalities suggest the diagnosis, which is verified by liver biopsy.

Treatment is with small frequent meals with a high carbohydrate content.

Further reading

Guthrie, R. A., Bustamante, S. and Paxson, C. L. (1979). Metabolic disorders. In *Van Leeuwen's Newborn Medicine*, Ed. by C. L. Paxon, p. 272. (Chicago; Year Book Medical Publishers)
Howell, R. R. (1972). The glycogen storage diseases. In *The Metabolic Basis of Inherited Disease*, Ed. by J. B. Stanbury, J. B. Wyngaarden and D. S. Fredrickson, 3rd edn., p. 155. (New York; McGraw-Hill)
Sinclair, L. (ed.) (1979). Hypoglycaemia. In *Metabolic Disease in Childhood*, p. 105. (Oxford; Blackwell Scientific Publications)

Case 69

Answers

1. X-linked nephrogenic diabetes insipidus (DI).
2. (a) Urine osmolarity.
   (b) Response to vasopressin (ADH) or desmopressin (DDAVP) on urine osmolarity.
   (c) Further family history of male children especially infant deaths.
   (d) Further history of polyuria and thirst in the patient and any other family member.
   (e) Plasma ADH when patient hyperosmolar.
3. (a) Low protein and sodium, high carbohydrate and fat diet.
   (b) Adequate water intake.
   (c) Hydrochlorothiazide with potassium supplements.

Discussion

This little boy is dehydrated, hypernatraemic, normokalaemic and markedly hyperosmolar although apparently still passing urine. Although gastroenteritis in an infant may result in hypernatraemic dehydration this is generally associated with injudicious feeds. This child is said to have been on clear fluids. The content is not mentioned, but this suggests that medical help has already been sought. The history of failure to thrive and repeated pyrexial episodes of unexplained aetiology suggests a metabolic or immune abnormality. Immune defects are rather unlikely since no specific infection has been found. In a child of 7 months who is already failing to thrive, this would be very unusual.

Hypernatraemia and dehydration may be caused by excessive salt intake when dehydrated — as mentioned above — too much water loss, or too much salt retention which is difficult to explain in the face of dehydration. The differential diagnosis is between DI, both hypothalamic and nephrogenic in origin, and congenital hyperaldosteronism. The latter is very rare but may produce severe growth retardation plus polydipsia, polyuria, intermittent paralysis, fatigue or muscular weakness, some of these symptoms resulting from potassium depletion. Serum sodium, pH and bicarbonate concentrations are all raised, potassium and chloride levels low. Hypertension always occurs secondary to the raised intravascular volume from sodium and water retention, and there may be cardiomegaly plus retinopathy.

No history is given of polyhydramnios in pregnancy, polydipsia or polyuria, but would probably be forthcoming if asked for. DI, both hypothalamic and nephrogenic in origin, may present in infancy with polyuria, polydipsia and dehydration. The initial clue to nephrogenic DI often is repeated episodes of unexplained fever. A family history of similar problems in males since it is usually x-linked would support the diagnosis. In both types of DI severe dehydration may present in infancy with constipation, vomiting and fever, resulting in marked failure to thrive because of inadequate calorie intake secondary to the severe thirst for water. In hypothalamic DI, hyperthermia, rapid weight loss and collapse are common in infancy. In both types severe dehydration may result in brain damage. In nephrogenic DI the severity of retardation is related to the age at which the diagnosis is made and therapy started. This is due not only to dehydration but also hypernatraemia. Hypernatraemia appears to be a fairly constant feature since maximum urine osmolarity is usually 80–150 mosmol. ℓ^{-1}. Any solute load such as sodium, chloride and urea thus require a large urine volume in which to be excreted. Nephrogenic DI should be suspected when there is persistently hypotonic urine in the face of clinical dehydration, or an elevated serum sodium or osmolarity. The critical test is the lack of rise in urine osmolarity in response to vasopressin (or the synthetic DDAVP) in this situation. Increased urine osmolarity would occur in hypothalamic DI. It is possible to measure plasma ADH by radio-immunoassay prior to giving DDAVP.

In nephrogenic diabetes insipidus, the distal tubules and collecting ducts are insensitive to ADH, thus diffusion of luminal water into the hypertonic medullary interstitium is markedly reduced. The exact reason for this is unknown and may involve various breaks in the pathway by which ADH increases the tubular permeability to water. This involves ATP dephosphorylation to cyclic AMP catalysed by adenyl cyclase and ADH. Inadequate production of cyclic AMP is not the final answer, however, since it is not reduced in all subjects studied. There are many other factors that influence this chain of events. These include: renal prostaglandins and drugs such as lithium, hypercalcaemia and hypokalaemia. The latter are both causes of polyuria. Primary polydipsia, (habit water drinking) can produce hypokalaemia and partial lack of tubular permeability to water. A prolonged water deprivation test may be required to show increasing urine osmolarity. Other causes of polyuria are caused by the primary defect being in the medullary solute gradient. Examples are: chronic renal failure, chronic obstructive nephropathy, medullary cystic disease, Fanconi's syndrome and interstitial nephropathy.

Treatment is aimed at (i) giving sufficient fluids and calories; (ii) reducing the solute load; and (iii) trying to reduce the urine volume. A diet high in carbohydrate and fat, but low in protein and salt (which increase the solute load) should be given, always with a high water intake. Diuretics, such as hydrochlorothiazide in combination with a low sodium intake, appear to reduce the urine volume by up to 50 per cent. The mechanism is not fully understood but it appears that together they produce a state of sodium depletion, which leads to a greater reabsorption of salt and water than normal in the proximal tubule. This alone appears to reduce the volume of fluid delivered to the loop of Henle and distal tubule. Potassium supplements will obviously be necessary. Indomethacin, as a prostaglandin inhibitor, is at present being assessed for its therapeutic role.

Hirschsprung's disease has been suggested as one of the differential diagnoses here. This could be true with the history of constipation and intermittent diarrhoea. Vomiting may occur secondary to partial intestinal obstruction. Severe dehydration would be most unlikely unless fulminant enterocolitis was present, in which case electrolyte losses should have occurred and hypernatraemia would not occur. A 7-month-old child who is failing to thrive owing to Hirschspring's disease would have moderate to severe disease and thus marked abdominal distension. In view of the symptoms, signs and investigations, a diagnosis of Hirschspring's disease cannot be justified.

Further reading

Hendricks, S. A. *et al.* (1981). Differential diagnosis of diabetes insipidus: use of DDAVP to terminate the 7 hour water deprivation test. *Journal of Pediatrics*, **98**, 244–246.

Koepp, P. (1979). Congenital nephrogenic diabetes insipidus (letter). *Archives of disease in childhood*, **54**, 807.

Stern, P. (1979). Nephrogenic defects of urinary concentration. In *Diseases of the Kidney*, Ed. by C. M. Edelmann, vol. **11**, pp. 978–993. (Philadelphia; Little, Brown)

Case 70

Answers

1. Pericarditis, acute.
2. (a) Bacterial secondary to chest infection, e.g. staphylococcal, streptococcal.
   (b) Viral, e.g. coxsackie A.
   (c) Tuberculosis.
3. (a) ECG.
   (b) Chest X-ray.
   (c) Ultrasound echocardiogram.
   (d) Blood culture.
   (e) Pericardial tap.
   (f) Viral studies.
   (g) Mantoux test.
   (h) Counter-current immunoelectrophoresis for *Haemophilus influenzae* and *Streptococcus pneumoniae*.
4. (a) Appropriate antibiotics.
   (b) Pericardiotomy.

Discussion

This patient presents with most of the classic symptoms and signs of acute pericarditis. These are: fever; pain which can be retrosternal (worse on lying down) but also referred to the neck or shoulder since the lower third of the pericardium is innervated by the phrenic nerve; dyspnoea; cough; paradoxial pulse and pericardial rub. Bacterial infections account for about 30 per cent of cases of acute pericarditis in the UK; the usual organisms are staphylococci, streptococci, pneumococci and *H. influenzae*. Most frequently it is caused by a spread from a pulmonary septic focus. This is the most likely explanation in this boy in view of the FBC which is highly suggestive of a bacterial infection, and signs in the chest consistent with right middle-lobe consolidation. Secondly, a viral cause is likely, and coxsackie viruses are most frequently isolated. This used to be labelled idiopathic pericarditis and accounts for a further 30 per cent of cases of acute pericarditis. Other viruses such as echo-, adeno- and EBV have been isolated.

Tuberculosis as a cause of acute pericarditis is rare in children except in the tropics where it should always be kept in mind. It usually spreads from hilar nodes or a lesion in the lung and this should be considered in this patient.

Rheumatic fever and post-pericardiotomy syndrome are the other main causes of acute pericarditis. These are particularly unlikely here. Pericarditis only occurs as part of a general carditis in rheumatic fever and is therefore almost always associated with an intracardiac murmur. Joint manifestations may precede it by many years.

Investigations are self-evident: ECG to show concave ST wave elevation and possibly T wave inversion; chest X-ray to show cardiomegaly with loss of the cardiac outline to a more spherical shape; echocardiogram (a reliable, non-invasive method of confirming the presence of a pericardial effusion); pericardial tap is mandatory in order to obtain fluid for microscopy and culture; blood culture in case of a septicaemia which is common in cases of bacterial aetiology. Other investigations mentioned are not urgent.

Active treatment with appropriate antibiotics is indicated in this child. Purulent pericarditis is usually treated with surgical drainage; fatalities are almost always due to failure to perform a surgical pericardiotomy.

Further reading

Benzing, G. and Kaplan, S. (1963). Purulent pericarditis. *American Journal of Diseases of Children*, **106**, 289.
Graham, G. and Rossi, A. (eds) (1980). *Heart Disease in Infants and Children*, p. 448. (London; Edward Arnold)
Spodick, D. H. (1971). Differential diagnosis of acute pericarditis. *Progress in Cardiovascular Disease*, **14**, 192.

Case 71

Answers

1. (a) Marfan's syndrome.
   (b) Homocystinuria.
2. (a) Increased urinary excretion of hydroxyproline in Marfan's syndrome.
   (b) Increased urinary excretion of homocystine.

Discussion

Five of the children attend the school yet only two are singled out for unwelcome attention. This suggests that there are visible abnormalities which may be inherited. The child is abnormally tall and has pectus excavatum. He also has ocular abnormalities including an episode of acute glaucoma and now retinal detachment. Two diseases which explain these findings are Marfan's syndrome and homocystinuria. Other differential diagnoses of excess height such as Kleinfelter's syndrome and juvenile acromegaly do not explain all the stigmata, especially the eye signs.

Marfan's syndrome is an autosomal dominant inherited disease with an incidence of 2–3 per 200 000 population. The biochemical abnormality involves mucopolysaccharide metabolism causing defects in connective tissue and excess urinary excretion of hydroxyproline.

The earliest sign may be the upward dislocation of the lens, which can occur congenitally. Lens dislocation in homocystinuria is downward and is never present at birth. Other ocular changes common to both diseases are myopia, glaucoma and retinal detachment.

Skeletal abnormalities include excess height, arachnodactyly, chest deformity, often pectus excavatum and spinal problems which may include kyphoscoliosis, hemivertebrae, vertebral fusion and spina bifida. The joints are hyperextensible — Steinberg's sign, extension of the opposed thumb past the ulnar border of the hand, is positive. The skeletal changes are thought to be due to generalized endochondral hyperplasia.

Severe cardiothoracic abnormalities may occur. The aorta and pulmonary artery may dilate with subsequent aneurysm formation and dissection. Valvular abnormalities include aortic and mitral incompetence. Congenital heart disease is rare, but has been described in association with Marfan's syndrome. Lesions described include Fallot's tetralogy, patent ductus arteriosus, stenosis of the aortic isthmus and ventricular septal defect.

Homocystinuria is a recessively inherited abnormality of amino acid metabolism due to a deficiency of cystathionine synthetase. Homocystine is an important intermediate in methionine metabolism which is included in protein synthesis. This may explain the connective tissue malfunction. Clinical features are manifest in three main areas: connective tissue, thrombotic phenomena and neuropsychiatric disturbances. A malar flush is common and telangiectases may occur at the edge of scar tissue. The hair is fair and sparse. Ocular changes include cataracts in addition to those already mentioned. Skeletal abnormalities include excess height with increased span, kyphoscoliosis and pectus excavatum. Generalized osteoporosis occurs which predisposes to spontaneous fractures. Joint mobility is reduced and Steinberg's sign is negative in contradistinction to Marfan's syndrome.

Thrombotic episodes occur in virtually all affected patients and no vessel is immune. Angina pectoris or sudden death may occur from involvement of the coronary arteries. Repeated cerebral thrombosis is a factor in the neuropsychiatric manifestations. 50 per cent only of sufferers have normal intelligence. It has been suggested that a schizoid personality is common in this disease.

Two varieties of homocystinuria are recognized, one pyridoxine sensitive the other pyridoxine resistant. The former may respond to pharmaceutical doses of vitamin B6. Both may be treated, with varying success, with a diet low in methionine but with added cystine.

Further reading

Gerritsen, T. and Waisman, H. A. (1972) Homocystinuria. In *The Metabolic Basis of Inherited Disease*, Ed. by J. B. Stanbury, J. B. Wyngaarden and D. S. Fredrickson, 3rd edn., p. 404. (New York; McGraw-Hill)

Rossi, E. (1980). Cardiomyopathies. In *Heart Disease in Infants and Children*, Ed. by C. Graham and E. Rossi, p. 466. (London; Edward Arnold)

Scriver, C. R. and Efron, M. L. (1972). Disorders of proline and hydroxyproline metabolism. In *The Metabolic Basis of Inherited Disease*, Ed. by J. B. Stanbury, J. B. Wyngaarden and J. B. Fredrickson, 3rd edn., p. 351. (New York; McGraw-Hill)

Sinclair, L. (ed.) (1979). Disorders of intermediary metabolism. In *Metabolic Disease in Childhood*, p. 434. (Oxford; Blackwell Scientific Publications)

Case 72

Answers

1. Isoimmune thrombocytopenia.
2. Platelet antibody studies on mother and child, particularly against father's platelets.
3. (a) Platelet transfusions, especially with mother's washed platelets.
   (b) Steroids.
   (c) Exchange transfusion.

Discussion

There are several causes of thrombocytopenia in a neonate such as: maternal idiopathic thrombocytopenic purpura (ITP), intrauterine infection, disseminated intravascular coagulopathy, sepsis, congenital thrombocytopenia or leukaemia and maternal drug ingestion. All of these may occur in one child, but three successive children with thrombocytopenia suggests a common process, the most likely being isoimmune thrombocytopenia. A mechanism similar to rhesus disease of the newborn operates where the mother has developed antibodies to a factor on the father's platelets which is present on the child's platelets. Thus mother's platelet count will be normal and antibody titres will not reveal a problem. The antibodies cross the placenta causing thrombocytopenia at birth, hopefully not so profound that intracerebral haemorrhage, the main danger, occurs. Following birth, thrombocytopenia will continue until the antibody is cleared from the blood.

Treatment must aim to tide the baby over the period of thrombocytopenia and secondly to reduce the amount of antibody. Platelet transfusions may be helpful, but these have a short life, will have to be repeated and may be destroyed by the antibodies present. Thus mother's washed platelets are the most logical source to use. Exchange transfusion with fresh blood should reduce the antibody load and thirdly steroids may be used as in idiopathic thrombocytopenic purpura. Although not proved in the latter condition, steroids are usually helpful in a definite immune process. They have been used in all three siblings.

Diagnosis is made by detecting platelet antibodies. This can be done specifically by taking the father's platelets and mixing them with serum from the mother and from the baby to obtain aggregation. Bone marrow aspiration will demonstrate normal red and white cell precursors with increased numbers of megakaryocytes. This would certainly support the theory of increased platelet turnover, in contrast to marrow depression, but does not demonstrate whether there is increased platelet destruction, or decreased budding of platelets from the megakaryocytes. Bone marrow aspiration is thus helpful but not diagnostic.

Further reading

Pearson, H. A., et al. (1964). Isoimmune neonatal thrombocytopenia purpura. Clinical and therapeutic considerations. *Blood*, **23**, 154.
Willoughby, M. L. N. (1977). Thrombocytopenia in the neomatal period. *Paediatric Haematology*, pp. 264–280. (Edinburgh; Churchill Livingstone)

Case 73

Answers

1. Ectopic ureter opening distal to the bladder.
2. (a) IVP.
   (b) Micturating cystourethrogram (MCU).
   (c) Ultrasound.
   (d) Aortogram.

Discussion

The history of this child is classic of a low-placed ectopic ureter, either in the lower urethra, vestibule or vagina. There is persistent dampness despite normal micturition at normal intervals. There are several other causes of persistent dribbling including neurogenic bladder, ectopic ureterocoele causing infravesical obstruction, and posterior urethral valves, but none are accompanied by normal micturition. Certain diagnosis can, however, be difficult. An IVP will demonstrate a non-opacified upper pole of the affected kidney, but as the renal remnant is often unable to concentrate any dye the ureter will not be delineated. A large, tortuous ureter may be demonstrated by ultrasound; occasionally a renal arteriogram or an aortogram can be used. It may be possible to detect a urethral opening on urethroscopy, but high vaginal openings are notoriously difficult to find. An MCU may demonstrate reflex into the ectopic ureter if the opening is in the bladder or upper urethra. If all fails an exploratory operation is indicated.

Treatment is by heminephrouretectomy or nephrouretectomy as the renal tissue drained by the ectopic ureter usually has poor or no function. Re-implantation has little to offer, therefore. The complete length of the ureter should be removed except in boys if there is involvement of the vas deferens and seminal vesicle.

Accessory ureteric buds arise cranial to the normal buds and, therefore, drain the upper renal moiety; however, the distal opening is always lower than that of the normal ureter and may involve the bladder neck, posterior urethra, wolffian or müllerian duct derivatives. If both ureters from a kidney are ectopic, that draining the upper moiety still drains to a lower point than the other. Ectopic ureters are subject to dilatation and reflux except for those opening into the trigone where there appears to be sufficient muscular tone to prevent reflux.

The mode of presentation depends on the positioning of the ureter and the sex of the child. The commonest ectopic position in females is in the bladder neck area. Incontinence is not a feature and presentation is severe, persistent or recurrent pyuria. If the opening is lower, infection is far less common and, characteristically, the child presents with persistent dribbling incontinence punctuated by normal micturition. Occasionally the child may be dry at night, probably due to a reservoir effect of the dilated ureter. Rarely, the child may have been completely dry before the onset of symptoms. This usually occurs when the ectopic opening is in the lower urethra; the musculature maintains continence until the ureter becomes dilated.

In males, the ectopic ureter may join the posterior urethra, ejaculatory duct or vas deferens. Incontinence is rarer than in the female, the presenting complaints commonly being severe pyuria or epididymitis. Often there is a single ectopic ureter draining the whole kidney which is dysplastic or ectopic itself. Diagnosis and treatment are as outlined above.

Further reading

Innes-Williams, D. (ed.) (1969). Ureteric duplications and ectopia. *Paediatric Urology*, p. 201. (London; Butterworths)

Johnston, J. H. and Mix, L. W. (1978). Indications for investigation of the urinary tract in the newborn. In *Neonatal Surgery*, Ed. by P. P. Rickham, J. Lister and I. M. Irving, 2nd edn., p. 555. (London; Butterworths)

Case 74

Answers

1. (a) *Mycoplasma pneumoniae* antibody titres.
   (b) *Mycoplasma pneumoniae* complement fixation test.
   (c) Cold agglutinin titre.
   (d) Viral antibodies.
   (e) Psittacosis and Q fever complement fixation titre.
2. (a) Erythromycin.
   (b) Tetracycline.

Discussion

This case history gives away the diagnosis by the classic history of *Mycoplasma pneumoniae* infection.

On reading the case history initially one thinks of tuberculosis, but the negative mantoux test result and lack of lymphocytosis in the peripheral blood and pleural fluid make this diagnosis most unlikely. An 'atypical' pneumonia in which there are clinical signs of lower respiratory tract infection associated with respiratory symptoms, but lack of response to the usual antibiotics employed such as ampicillin, is usually caused by *Mycoplasma pneumoniae* but other organisms that should be considered are viruses, especially the adenovirus, *Chlamydia psittaci*, i.e. psittacosis, and *Coxiella burnetii*, i.e. Q fever pneumonia.

Mycoplasma infections are most frequent in school-age children. However, in children under 5, when screened, many asymptomatic infections have been found. Pneumonic disease in the older age groups may be an expression of increasing host immune response to the organism, and many of the complications may result through immunological mechanisms. The incubation period is about 12–14 days. The first symptoms are 'flu like' with headache, fever, chills, malaise and anorexia followed by a sore throat and dry cough.

Other symptoms include nasal discharge, vomiting, abdominal pain, earache, and non-specific skin rashes. Mucoid sputum may be produced later, and when seen in hospital a large number of patients have failed to respond to antibiotics.

Physical signs are very variable. Fever is usual, but chest signs can be lobar, unilateral, bilateral or generalized, and generally consist both of crepitations and less frequently of rhonchi. Occasionally a pleural effusion may be present. Pharyngeal oedema, skin rashes, tender cervical lymph nodes, otitis media and conjunctivitis may also be present.

The chest X-ray is also variable with either a lobar or multifocal consolidation. Quite frequently the chest X-ray changes are mild in comparison with the physical findings and vice versa. If decubitus views are taken, pleural effusions are found in up to a quarter of cases. They are exudates, with no organisms on Gram's stain or culture, but with WBC counts from 5 to 6000 $\times$ 10^9. ℓ^{-1}. The peripheral WBC count is usually normal with an absolute neutrophilia as in this case. Cold agglutinins occur in about 50 per cent of cases but are less common in children than adults. If present with a respiratory infection, it is highly suggestive of mycoplasma although cold agglutinins are also present in infectious mononucleosis, adenovirus and other infections. There is a simple cold agglutinin screening test (CAST) which can be done at the bedside. This consists of mixing 50/50 blood and citrate together in a prothrombin tube, and placing it in a deep-freezer compartment for a few minutes. On removal obvious agglutination can be seen on the wall of the tube if the test is positive and disappears on warming. Confirmation with antibody titres done by indirect immunofluorescence is a prolonged method; complement fixation titres on acute and convalescent serum showing a fourfold rise or more, or a single titre of 1:64, is highly suggestive; and lastly isolation of *M. pneumoniae* from sputum is possible but difficult.

Differential diagnosis from psittacosis, which may present in a very similar fashion to mycoplasma with diffuse or patchy chest X-ray changes, should be made with rise in complement fixing antibodies, isolation of the chlamydial organism if possible and a history of exposure to birds. Q fever principally affects the lungs and should be looked for by a rise in antibody titre, but complement fixing or agglutination tests are more reliable. The Weil–Felix reaction was used previously to look for rickettsial infection. Legionnaire's disease should be considered in the differential diagnosis of severe lobar pneumonia.

Viral infections may be diagnosed by increase in specific antibody titres on paired serum samples approximately 2 weeks apart, if these are available.

Reported complications of mycoplasma infections are many and variable. These include bullous myringitis, Stevens–Johnson syndrome, adult respiratory distress syndrome, haemolytic anaemia, myocarditis, Guillain–Barré syndrome, poliomyelitis-like syndrome, meningitis, arthritis, glomerulonephritis, genital disease and sterility.

Treatment is usually with erythromycin in children but tetracycline may be used in children over 12 years when the danger of permanently staining the teeth is over.

Further reading

Fernald, G. W., *et al.* (1979). Respiratory infections due to *Mycoplasma pneumoniae* in infants and children. *Pediatrics*, **55**, 327–335.

Lane, D. J. (1979). Pneumonia. *Medicine*, Series 3, **23**, 1177–1182.

Levine, D. P. and Lerner, A. M. (1978). The clinical spectrum of *Mycoplasma pneumoniae* infection. *Medical Clinics of North America*, **62**, 961–978.

McFarlane, J. T., *et al.* (1979). Rapid diagnosis of *Mycoplasma pneumoniae* infection: A reminder (letter). *British Medical Journal*, **i**, 124.

Pumarola, A., *et al.* (1979). Mycoplasma pneumoniae infections. *Paediatrician*, **8**, 56–64.

Stevens, D., *et al.* (1978). *Mycoplasma pneumoniae* infections in children. *Archives of Disease in Childhood*, **53**, 38–42.

Case 75

Answers

1. (a) Establishment of an airway.
   (b) Intravenous antibiotics.
2. (a) Blood gases.
   (b) Blood cultures.

(c) X-ray of lateral neck.
(d) Bacterial throat swabs.

Discussion

This child presents clinically with acute epiglottitis which is usually caused by *Haemophilus influenzae* type B. The history is short and he presents as a toxic, pyrexial child with respiratory embarrassment, cyanosis from hypoxia and restlessness from hypercapnia. The immediate action is to ensure the patency of the airway. Acute epiglottitis is a rapidly progressive, potentially lethal disease so speed in establishing an airway is of paramount importance. The child may be intubated by an experienced anaesthetist, preferably with an Ear, Nose and Throat surgeon in attendance, or an elective tracheostomy performed. The child is then given humidified air to breathe. Once the airway is established the appropriate intravenous antibiotics are given and blood gases taken to assess the acid–base balance. There is still debate as to the efficacy of steroids in reducing tissue oedema.

Acute epiglottitis is the most likely diagnosis and may be confirmed by appropriate investigation. However, other diagnoses should be considered.

Viral infection of the respiratory tree — such as acute laryngitis, laryngotracheitis or laryngotracheobronchitis — usually has a longer history, but laryngotracheobronchitis may present acutely and, if the oedema extends distally, the respiratory embarrassment may not be relieved by intubation. Implicated viruses are parainfluenza, ECHO viruses, respiratory syncitial virus and coxsackie viruses. At laryngoscopy the epiglottis is normal, but there is marked oedema distally. Treatment is also by intubation if indicated or by humidified air. Antibiotics are not indicated. Occasionally *Haemophilus influenzae* can cause laryngotracheobronchitis. If this is considered, appropriate antibiotics should be started.

Inhaled foreign bodies may impact in the glottis and cause immediate stridor which is worsened by subsequent oedema or mucosal haemorrhage. This would not, however, produce such a high pyrexia. Differentration is often possible on lateral neck X-ray.

Angioneurotic oedema may present rapidly after an inhaled or ingested allergen. No rash indicating urticaria was noted, although oedema may occur without a peripheral rash. At laryngoscopy the tissues are pale and oedematous rather than brilliant red in the infective states. Treatment is with subcutaneous adrenaline or intravenous hydrocortisone and antihistamines.

Further reading

Krugman, S. and Katz, S. L. (eds) (1982). Acute respiratory infections. Clinical syndromes. In *Infectious Diseases of Children*, 7th edn., p. 288. (St. Louis; C. V. Mosky)

Milner, A. and Buffin, J. T. (1979). Upper airways obstruction. In *Paediatric Emergencies*, Ed. by J. A. Black. p. 218. (London; Butterworths)

Williams, H. E. and Phelan, P. D. (1975). Clinical patterns of acute respiratory infection. In *Respiratory Illness in Children*, Ed. by H. E. Williams and P. D. Phelan, pp. 26-35. (Oxford; Blackwell Scientific Publications)

Case 76

Answers

1. ECG.
2. Aortic stenosis.
3. (a) Echocardiography.
   (b) Cardiac catheterization.

Discussion

This previously healthy child presents with a sudden transient loss of consciousness with no neurological sequelae. This argues against a toxic or infective encephalopathy. The immediate thought, therefore, may be of a simple faint. The weather was hot, the episode short, the blood pressure marginally low and there were no sequelae. However, the presence of a diastolic murmur is pathological and the combination of such a murmur, a systolic murmur, a soft second sound and a marginally low blood pressure suggests aortic stenosis with incompetence. An ECG would show left ventricular hypertrophy with large R and S waves in the left and right leads, respectively. Left-sided strain is indicated by ST depression with or without T wave inversion over the left chest leads.

Echocardigraphy is a useful non-invasive technique for viewing the aortic valve and outflow tract. However, as the stenosis was sufficiently severe to cause cerebral hypoxia, cardiac catheterization is indicated to determine the pressure gradient across the aortic valve.

Aortic stenosis constitutes 5 per cent of cardiac malformations and is three times more prevalent in males than females. The obstruction may be supravalvular, valvular or subvalvular. Valvular may be either fused cusps or an abnormal bicuspid valve, as in this child. Subvalvular may be either discrete, such as a fibrous ring, or a diffuse obstructive cardiomyopathy — hypertrophic obstructive cardiomyopathy (HOCM).

Many children are symptomless, even with moderately severe stenosis. Others may have dyspnoea on exertion or cerebral hypoxia causing loss of consciousness. Aortic stenosis is always quoted as one of the causes of childhood angina, but chest pain occurs in the minority of cases.

Examination may reveal jerky pulses in HOCM or an anacrotic pulse in the other types. The systolic blood pressure may be reduced, but often not strikingly so. The second heart sound may be soft or have reversed splitting. The ejection systolic murmur may be heard at the apex, base, or left sternal edge. A diastolic murmur may be from aortic stenosis or secondary to mitral regurgitation accompanying HOCM. An early systolic click may be heard at the apex. In severe disease a double atrial beat may be felt.

Surgery is indicated by the presence of chest pain, loss of consciousness, ST depression on an ECG and a pressure gradient in excess of 55 mmHg across the stenotic valve.

Sadly, this congenital anomaly is a cause of sudden death and it is extremely difficult to define the 'at risk' population. There is usually no family history, except occasionally in HOCM which can have an autosomal dominent inheritance, and the children are often symptomless.

Further reading

Banoldi, G. (1982). Sudden death. In *The Heart*, Ed. by J. Willis Hurst, 5th edn., p. 591. (New York; McGraw-Hill)

Rackley, C. E., Edwards, J. E., Karp, R. B. and Kirklin, J. W. (1982). Aortic valve disease. In *The Heart*, Ed. by J. Willis Hurst, 5th edn., p. 863. (New York; McGraw-Hill)

Roberts, W. C., Mason, D. T., Eugle, M. A. and Cohn, L. H. (eds) (1982). Valvular heart disease. In *Cardiology*, p. 230. (New York; Yorke Medical Books)

Weber, J. W. (1980). Congenital aortic stenosis. In *Heart Disease in Infants and Children*, Ed. by G. Graham and E. Rossi, p. 259. (London; Edward Arnold)

Case 77

Answers

1. Pulmonary atresia with an intact ventricular septum.
2. (a) Echocardiography.
   (b) Cardiac catheterization.
   (c) Cardiac angiography.

Discussion

This infant has a ductus arteriosus dependent cardiac lesion. The indomethacin infusion caused a partial closure of the duct. This caused a deep cyanosis which was reversed by prostaglandin E. Having partially closed the duct, the wisdom of then placing the child in oxygen, with the possibility of further ductal closure, is debatable. The ventricular septum must be intact and there must also be a right-to-left shunt. If there was a left-to-right shunt, one would expect right ventricle dominance on the ECG and plethoric lung fields. The most common possibilities, therefore, are transposition of the great vessels and tricuspid of pulmonary atresia, or severe pin-hole stenosis.

The chest X-ray was reported as oligaemic, which is against transposition; also the adult pattern is not typical of a transposition ECG. A single second sound may be heard, however.

The findings are also not entirely consistent with tricuspid atresia. The chest X-ray findings can be similar, the second sound may be single, but the ECG classically displays a left axis deviation. The most likely diagnosis is therefore, pulmonary atresia or severe stenosis, with an intact ventricular septum.

Pulmonary atresia is rare, accounting for only 1 per cent of congenital cardiac lesions. The atresia is usually valvular only but may occasionally be infundibular. There are two main varieties. The more common (80–85 per cent) have a small right ventricle associated with a hypoplastic tricuspid valve; the rest have a normal or large right ventricle, often associated with tricuspid incompetence. Either type may have an intact or perforated ventricular septum. If the septum is intact, pulmonary flow is via a patent ductus arteriosus and the bronchial vessels.

Pulmonary atresia has developmental consequences. The aorta does not taper smoothly and does not have an isthmal narrowing or post-ductal dilatation, the pulmonary artery is very small and there is a reversal of flow in the ductus arteriosus. If the ductus is small, marked cyanosis occurs; if large, cyanosis may be absent. On consultation, the first heart sound is invariably single if the right ventricle and tricuspid valve are small. There may be a soft mid-systolic murmur from the ductus arteriosus. With a large right ventricle, the first sound may also be single and the systolic murmurs are consequent on the anatomy of the tricuspid valve. The second heart sound is obviously single. The ECG may be the key to diagnosis as the combination of cyanosis with left ventricular dominance is highly suggestive of pulmonary atresia. There is also a normal right-sided axis.

The cardiac silhouette is usually normal in the neonatal period, but the left ventricle and right atrium rapidly enlarge as does the aorta.

The echocardiogram is useful for determining chamber and vessel size and the exact anatomy can be demonstrated by cardiac angiography.

The prognosis is poor — up to 50 per cent of infants die within the first month of life. Surgical treatment is possible and approaches include the formation of a pulmonary systemic anastomosis, reconstruction of the pulmonary outflow tract or the construction of an external conduit from the right atrium or ventricle to the pulmonary artery.

Further reading

Marriott, H. J. K. (ed.) (1977). The Heart. In *Childhood and Congenital Lesions*, 6th edn., p. 284. (Baltimore; Williams and Wilkins)

Oran, S. (ed.) (1981). Congenital heart disease. In *Clinical Heart Disease*, 3rd edn., p. 512. (London; William Heinemann Books)

Perloff, J. K. (ed.) (1978). Pulmonary atresia with intact ventricular septum. In *Clinical Recognition of Congenital Heart Disease*, 2nd edn., p. 604. (Philadelphia; W. B. Saunders)

Index

Note: Page numbers in *italics* refer to those pages on which the case presentation appears, but where the disorder is not named. 'vs' denotes differential diagnosis.

Abdominal mass, 124, 156
  inguinal, *42*, 165
  in obstructed infected kidney, 124
Abdominal pain, *see* Pain, abdominal
Abscess,
  anal, 33
  cerebral, *56–57*, 145, 183–184
  'cold', on chest wall, 33, 152
  pelvic appendix, *55–56*, 182
  vas deferens, inguinal mass, 165
Achalasia, of cardia, 229
Acid maltase deficiency, 215
Acidosis,
  in galactosaemia, fructosaemia, 199, 200
  in organic acidurias, 198
  in Von Gierke's disease, *96*, 231
  lactic, 198
  renal tubular, 178, 194
Acute lymphoblastic leukaemia (ALL), *29–30*, 145–147
Adenitis, mesenteric, 182
Adenoids, enlarged, *79–80*, 213
Adrenal haemorrhage, 114
Adrenal hyperplasia, congenital, *20*, 114, 135–137
Adrenal hypoplasia, congenital, *3*, 113–114
Agglutinins, cold, 243
Aggression, *66*, 194
Airway establishment, in acute epiglottitis, 245
Aldosterone deficiency, 113, 114
Alkaline phosphatase, in rickets, *12*, 125
Alpha-fetoprotein, in neuroblastoma, 129
1-Alphahydroxycholecalciferol, 178
δ-Aminolevulinic acid, 196
Ammonia, blood,
  in organic acidurias, 198
  in Reye's syndrome, 120
Amphotericin, in aspergillus infections, 154
Anaemia
  aplastic, *29–30*, 146
  hypochromic microcytic, 168, 186
  in G6PD deficiency, *93*, 227
  in haemolytic uraemic syndrome, 158
  in lead encephalopathy, 121, 122
  in sickle-cell disease, *2*, 109
  microangiopathic haemolytic, *36*, 157–158
Androgen production defects, 136
Angioneurotic oedema, 245
Antenatal diagnosis,
  cystic fibrosis, 185
  β-thalassaemia, 168
Antibiotics,
  blood-brain barrier permeable, 124
  in acute pericarditis, 236
  in endocarditis, atrioventricular shunt, 174–175
  in immune deficiency, 224
  in obstructed infected kidney, 123–124
  in pneumococcal meningitis, *14*, 128
Anticonvulsant therapy, rickets with, *11*, 125
Antidepressants,
  drug abuse with, *21*, *23*, 137, 140
  in migraine, 208
Anti-diuretic hormone (ADH),
  action, development, 222
  inappropriate secretion, 151, 161
  in hypothalamic diabetes insipidus, 117, 233
  in nephrogenic diabetes insipidus, 233–234
  response,
    in chronic renal failure, 117
    in nephrogenic diabetes insipidus, 233
Anti-nuclear factor,
  in chronic active hepatitis, 212
  in connective tissue syndromes, 203
  in juvenile rheumatoid arthritis, 110
Anti-streptolysin 'O' titre (ASOT), 110
α₁-Antitrypsin, 226
  deficiency, 212, 225, 226
Aortic stenosis, *105–106*, 246–247
Apnoea,
  of prematurity, *30*, 149
  in Von Gierke's disease, *95*, 231
Appendicitis, acute, 182

251

Appendix, pelvic, abscess, *55–56*, 182
Arteritis, in tuberculous meningitis, 161
Arthritis,
  juvenile chronic, 116, 147
  monoarticular, 1, 109, 115
  pauciarticular, 110
  rheumatoid, 110
  septic, 110, 111
  tuberculous, 115
Ascaris lumbricoides, 192
Ascaris suum, 192
Aspergillus, *33–34*, 152–154
Astrocytoma, *71–73*, 203–204, 205, 218
Ataxia, in astrocytomas, 204
Atrioventricular shunt, 48, 174

Bacterial infections, (*see also* Infections;
    individual infections)
  in acute pericarditis, 236
  in chronic granulomatous disease, 153
  in subdural empyema, 184
Behavioural disturbances, 78
  in acute intermittent porphyria, *66*, 195, 196
  in subacute sclerosing
    panencephalitis, *12–13*, 126
Bicarbonate renal threshold, 194
Biliary atresia,
  congenital, 225
  postnatal extrahepatic, *91*, 225
Bilirubin, determinations in jaundice, 199
Bite cells, 93, 227
Bladder, ectopic ureter opening distal
    to, *101–102*, 240–241
Bleeding, *see also* Haemorrhage
  haemoglobin drop, in premature
    infant, 135
  rectal, 61, 189
  upper intestinal, 189
  vaginal, 35, 155
Blind loop syndrome, 143
Blood transfusion,
  exchange, in isoimmune thrombo-
    cytopenia, 239
  in β-thalassaemia major, 169
Bone,
  age, assessment, 113
  aseptic necrosis, 109
  cysts, benign, 116
  fibrous dysplasia of, 156
  malignancies, 116

metastases, in neuroblastoma, 130
pain, 130, 146
Bone marrow, aspiration,
  in isoimmune thrombocytopenia, 240
  in leukaemia, 146, 203
Bowel,
  duplication cyst, 142–143
  malrotation, *25–27*, 142
Brain-stem astrocytoma, 204
Breath-holding episodes, 53, 179
Bronchiectasis, 209, 210
Bronchiolitis, 210
Bronchitis, wheezy, 62, 190
Bronchoscopy,
  in tracheo-oesophageal fistula, 230
  removal of foreign object, 190–191

Caeruloplasmin, 212
Café au lait spots, 35, 155–156
Calcification, intracerebral, 206
Calcinosis, 202
Campylobacter infections, 173, 219
Carbamazepine, ingestion, *59–60*, 187–188
Carcinoembryonic antigen, 129
Cardiac catheterization, 80
  in aortic stenosis, 246–247
  in pulmonary atresia, 249
  in right ventricular hypertrophy, 80, 213
Cardiac muscle, digoxin, xanthines
    effect, 216
Cardiomyopathy, hypertrophic
    obstructive, 247
Cardiothoracic abnormalities, in
    Marfan's syndrome, 237–238
Carotid angiography, 144
Catheterization,
  cardiac, (*see* Cardiac catheterization)
  in pelvic appendix abscess, 181, 182
Central core disease, 214
Central nervous system malignancy,
    50–51, 71–73, 175–176, 204, 205
Cerebellum,
  abscess, *56–57*, 183–184
  astrocytoma, 205
  haemorrhage, 144
  oedema, *57*, 171, 183
  sclerosis, 179
  space-occupying lesion, *71–73*, 204
  thrombosis, superficial venous, 183
  tumours, 145

convulsions in, 122
  precocious puberty, 156
Cerebral artery, left middle, occlusion, 27–28, 144
Cerebrospinal fluid (CSF),
  count, in tuberculous meningitis, 160
  protein, in Guillain-Barré syndrome, 220
Chédiak-Higashi syndrome, 154
Chemotaxis, defects, 153
Chest infections, (see also Respiratory tract infections)
  recurrent, 94, 229
Chickenpox,
  complications, 182
  paresis after, 31, 150–151
Child abuse, 21–22, 39, 137–138, 162
Chloramphenicol, in typhoid, 219
1α-Cholecalciferol, 194
25-OH Cholecalciferol, 177, 178
Choroidoretinitis, 206
Chronic granulomatous disease (CGD), 33–34, 82, 152–154, 223
Cineradiography, 230
Cirrhosis,
  in α_1-antitrypsin deficiency, 212, 226
  in Wilson's disease, 212
Clotting abnormality, 79, 211
Coeliac disease, 173, 186
Cold agglutinin screening test (CAST), 243
Collodion patches, 202
Coma, 119
  in aortic stenosis, 105, 246
  in drug poisoning, 21–22, 22, 137, 139–140
  in lead encephalopathy, 8, 121
  in Reye's syndrome, 7, 119
Computer assisted tomography (CT) scan,
  in extension of subdural empyema, 183
  in herpes encephalitis, 151
  in space-occupying lesion, 113, 160
Congenital adrenal hyperplasia (CAH), 20, 114, 135–137
Congenital adrenal hypoplasia, 3, 113–114
Congenital heart disease, 248
  aortic stenosis, 105–106, 246–247
  in Marfan's syndrome, 238
  pulmonary atresia, 107–108, 248–249

Connective tissue syndrome, 203
Constipation,
  in diabetes insipidus, 97, 233
  in Fanconi syndrome, 64, 193
  in giardiasis, 47, 173
  in Hirschsprung's disease, 182, 234
Constitutional pubertal and growth delay, 112
Convulsions,
  in cerebral tumours, 122
  in drug abuse, 21–22, 137
  in hyponatraemia, 89, 222
  in lead encephalopathy, 8, 121
  in tuberculous meningitis, 159
Coombs' test, 228
Coproporphyrinogen, 196
Corneal reflex, absent, 54, 179
Cor pulmonale, 82, 186
Coryza,
  frontal sinusitis after, 56–57, 183
  in Perthe's disease, 4
Co-trimoxazole, in typhoid, 219
Cough,
  in chronic suppurative lung disease, 75–76, 209
  in inhalation of foreign object, 62–63, 190
  in *Mycoplasma pneumoniae* infection, 103, 243
  in tracheo-oesophageal fistula, 94, 229
  in typhoid, 85, 219
  paroxysmal, in cystic fibrosis, 58, 185
  with feeding, causes, 94, 229
Cows' milk intolerance, 186
  vs. congenital adrenal hypoplasia, 114
  vs. cystic fibrosis, 186
  vs. pyloric stenosis, 197–198
Coxsackie virus, in pericarditis, 236
Cranial nerve palsy,
  VIth,
    in disseminated CNS malignancy, 50, 176–177
    in pseudotumour cerebri, 171
  in tuberculous meningitis, 161
  in viral encephalitis, 160
Creatine phosphokinase (CPK),
  in limb-girdle muscular dystrophy, 214
  in polymyositis, 215
Crohn's disease, 61, 111, 182, 189
Cyanosis,
  in acute epiglottitis, 104, 245

Cyanosis – *continued*
  in pulmonary atresia, *107*, 249
  with enlarged adenoids, tonsils, *79–80*, 213
Cyclic AMP, 216, 234
Cystic fibrosis, *58*, 185–186, 209–210
Cystinosis, 194–195
Cytomegalovirus (CMV) infection, 206, 207

Dactylitis, in sickle-cell disease, 109
Dehydration, 233
  in diabetes insipidus, *97*, 232–233
Depression, drug abuse with, *21, 23*, 137, 140
Dermatitis herpetiformis, 141
Dermatomyositis, *70–71*, 202
Desferrioxamine, 169
Desmopressin (DDAVP), 233
Diabetes insipidus, 117
  hypothalamic, 117, 233
    aetiology, 118
    idiopathic, 118
    vs. psychogenic polydipsia, 117–118
  in Hand-Schüller-Christian disease, *40*, 163
  nephrogenic, 117, 233
    X-linked, *96–98*, 232–234
Diabetes mellitus, 117
  Somogyi effect, *18*, 132–133
  vs. psychogenic polydipsia, 117
Diarrhoea,
  bloody, 189
  in Crohn's disease, 189
  in galactosaemia, *69*, 199, 200
  in neuroblastoma, *15*, 129
Diencephalic syndrome (*see* Hypothalamic tumour)
Diet,
  in fructosaemia, 201
  in galactosaemia, 200–201
  in nephrogenic diabetes insipidus, 234
  in Von Gierke's disease, 231
Digoxin, 82, 216
1α-Dihydroxycalciferol, 178
Diphtheria, 221
Disseminated intravascular coagulation (DIC), 158
Diuretics, in diabetes insipidus, 234
DMSA renal scan, 124

Down's syndrome, 73
Drowning, fresh-water, 139
Drugs, (*see also individual drugs*)
  in G6PD deficiency, 227
  intoxication, 119, 123
    non-accidental, *21–22*, 137–138
    peripheral neuropathy, 221
    self-, *23–24, 59–60*, 140, 187–188
    vs. tuberculous meningitis, 161
Ductus arteriosus, in pulmonary atresia, 248, 249
  patent, 107
Duplication cyst, 142–143
Dysautonomia, familial, *53–54*, 179–180
Dysentery, Shigella, 219
Dyspnoea,
  in acute pericarditis, *98*, 235
  in aortic stenosis, 247
  in chronic granulomatous disease, *33*, 152
  in extrahepatic biliary atresia, *91*

Echocardiography, 246, 249
Eisenmenger's syndrome, 213
Electrocardiogram, (ECG),
  in acute pericarditis, 236
  in aortic stenosis, 246
  in pulmonary atresia, 249
Electroencephalogram (EEG),
  in drug poisoning, *22*, 140
  in migraine, 208
  in varicella encephalitis, 151
Electrolytes, in fresh-water drowning, 139
Embolism, middle cerebral artery, 144
Emotional disturbance, 118 (*see also* Behavioural disturbances)
Empyema, subdural, 183, 184
Encephalitis,
  acute hemiplegia, 144
  herpes, 151, 171
  post-infectious, 151
  varicella, *31–32*, 150–151
  viral, 122, 160, 171
Encephalopathy,
  acute, causes, 221
  hepatic, 212
  lead, *see* Lead encephalopathy
Endocarditis, subacute bacterial, 174
Enteritis,
  regional, 111
  tuberculous, 189

Enterocolitis, fulminant, 234
Enuresis, 77, 101–102, 240–241
Eosinophilia,
　causes, 191
　pulmonary, 191–192
　tropical, *63–64*, 192
Eosinophilic granuloma, 163–164
Ependymoma, 176
Epiglottitis, acute, *104–105*, 245
Epilepsy, temporal lobe, 66, 195
　vs. migraine, 208
Ergotamine, 208
Erythema multiforme, *24–25*, 141
Erythromycin, in mycoplasma infections, 244
Ethamsylate, 167

Failure to thrive,
　in chronic granulomatous disease, *33*, 152
　in diabetes insipidus, *97*, 233
　in Fanconi syndrome, *64*, 192
　in SCID, *90*, 223, 224
　in vitamin-D resistant rickets, *51*
　with hypothalamic tumour, *83–84*, 217–218
Fanconi syndrome, *64–65*, 193–195, 200
　causes, 193, 194
　vs. galactosaemia, fructosaemia, 200
Favism, 227
Femoral epiphysis, ischaemic necrosis, 115
Femoral head,
　aseptic necrosis, 109
　in Perthes' disease, 115
Fibrin thrombi, in HUS, 158
Fibrous dysplasia, 156
Fistula,
　-in-ano, 189
　perianal, 189
Fluorescent spot test, 228
Folate deficiency, 186
Food allergy, 173
Foreign body, inhalation, *62–63*, 190–191
　vs. acute epiglottitis, 245
Fracture,
　femur, 39, 162
　multiple, child abuse, 162
　spiral, 162
　transverse, 162
Free erythrocyte protoporphyrin (FEP), 122

Frontal sinus, infection, *56–57*, 183
Fructokinase deficiency, 201
Fructosaemia, 200, 201, 225
Fructose-1-phosphate aldolase deficiency, 201

Gait,
　in limb-girdle muscular dystrophy, *81*, 214
　in subacute sclerosing panencephalitis, *13*, 126
　unsteady, cerebellar lesion, 204
Galactokinase deficiency, 200
Galactosaemia, 200–201, 225
Galactose-1-phosphate uridyl transferase deficiency, 200
Galactosuria, 200
Gastroenteritis,
　hypernatraemia in, 232
　lactose intolerance induced by, 186
Gastro-oesophageal reflux, 198
Genitalia, ambiguous, *20*, 135–137
Giardiasis, *47–48*, 172–173, 219
Glaucoma, 99, 237
Globin chains in β-thalassaemia, 168
Glucose-6-phosphatase deficiency, 231
Glucose-6-phosphate dehydrogenase (G6PD) deficiency, *92–93*, 134, 227–228
Gluten-free diet, 186
Glycogenosis,
　type I, *95–96*, 231
　type II, 215
Glycosuria, Somogyi effect, *18*, 133
Gonadotrophin deficiency, 112
Gonadotrophin-secreting tumours, 156–157
Graft-versus-host (GVH) reaction, 224
Granuloma, eosinophilic, 163–164
Growth delay, 2, 112
　constitutional pubertal and, 112
Growth hormone deficiency, 113, 163
Guillain-Barré syndrome,
　vs. poliomyelitis, 220
　vs. varicella encephalitis, 150

Haematoma, subdural, 139, 145
Haemoglobin,
　drop, in premature infant, *19*, 134
　in β-thalassaemia, 168
　in vitamin E deficiency, *19*, 134
Haemoglobin A, 168

Haemoglobin A_2, 168
Haemoglobin C disease, 109
Haemoglobin D, 109
Haemoglobin F, 168
Haemoglobinuria,
   in G6PD deficiency, *92*, 227
   paroxysmal cold, 228
   paroxysmal nocturnal, 228
Haemolysis,
   autoimmune, 227
   in G6PD deficiency, *92–93*, 227–228
   intravascular, causes, 228
   secondary to vitamin E deficiency, *19*, 134
Haemolytic uraemic syndrome (HUS), *36*, 157–159
Haemophilus influenzae type B, 245
Haemoptysis, 76, 209
Haemorrhage, (*see also* Bleeding)
   adrenal, 114
   'boat-shaped', retinal, 175
   cerebral, 144
   intraventricular (IVH), *43*, 149, 166
      categories, 166
   pulmonary, 166
   'splinter', 175
   subarachnoid, 139, 144
   subdural, 139, 145, 170
   sub-hyaloid, 139
Hallervorden-Spatz disease, 127
Halothane hepatitis, 211
Hand-Schüller-Christian disease, (*see* Histiocytosis X)
Haptoglobins, 228
Headaches, 2
   hypothalamic/pituitary space-occupying lesion, 112
   in astrocytoma, medulloblastoma, *71–73*, 203–205
   in migraine, 187
   in *Mycoplasma pneumoniae* infection, *103*, 243
   in pseudotumour cerebri, *45*
   in typhoid, *85*, 219
Head injury, 139, 170
Heart, murmurs, 106, 247, 249
Heart disease, congenital (*see* Congenital heart disease)
Heinz bodies, 227
Hemiplegia, acute, *27–28*, 143–145
   aetiology, 144
   in subdural empyema, *57*, 183

Hemithorax, transillumination, 166
Henle, loop of, neonatal, 222
Henoch-Schönlein purpura, 109
   vs. haemolytic uraemic syndrome, 158, 159
Hepatic portoenterostomy, 226
Hepatitis,
   acute, 211
   chronic active, 212
   conjugated hyperbilirubinaemia, 225
   halothane, 211
   infectious, 47, 173
   neonatal, 200
   non-A, non-B, 211
Hepatitis B, in aplastic anaemia, 147
Hepatosplenomegaly, 223
   in Von Gierke's disease, 231
Hernia,
   congenital inguinal, 165
   hiatus, 198, 229
   strangulated, 165
Herpes encephalitis, 151
Herpes hominis infection, 206
Herpes simplex infections, 144
Hiatus hernia, 198, 229
Hip,
   in Perthe's disease, *4*, 115
   transient synovitis, recurrent, 115
Hirschsprung's disease, 173
   vs. nephrogenic diabetes insipidus, 234
   vs. pelvic appendix abscess, 182
Histiocytosis X, *40–41*, 163–164
HLA, in juvenile rheumatoid arthritis, 110
Homocystine excretion, 238
Homocystinuria, *99–100*, 237–238
Horner's syndrome, 129
Human chorionic gonadotrophin, 113
Huntington's chorea, 126
Hydrocephalus,
   in astrocytoma, 204, 218
   in hypothalamic tumour, 217, 218
   in tuberculous meningitis, 161
   otitic, 170
Hydrochlorothiazide, 195, 234
Hydrogen breath tests, 186
Hydrogen peroxide, 153
Hydronephrosis,
   bilateral, 124
   right, infected, *9*, 123–124
17-Hydroxylase deficiency, 136
21-Hydroxylase deficiency, 136

17-Hydroxyprogesterone, 136
Hydroxyproline excretion, 237
3β-Hydroxysteroid dehydrogenase deficiency, 136
Hyperaldosteronism, congenital, 233
Hyperammonaemia, 198
Hyperbilirubinaemia, conjugated, 225
Hypercalciuria, in Fanconi syndrome, 194
Hypercapnia,
  enlarged tonsils, adenoids, *79–80*, 213
  in acute epiglottitis, *104*, 245
Hypercoagulability, 132
Hyperglycinaemia, 198
Hyperkalaemia, 113
Hyperlipidaemia, 231
Hypernatraemia, *96–98*, 232–234
Hyperparathyroidism, secondary, 125
Hyperphosphaturia, 194
Hyperreflexia, 119
  in Reye's syndrome, 119, 120
Hypertension,
  benign intracranial, *45–46*, 170–172
  cerebral haemorrhage with, 144
  in 17-hydroxylase deficiency, 136
  pulmonary, *80*, 213
Hyperthyroidism, 112, 218
Hypertrophic obstructive cardiomyopathy (HOCM), 247
Hyperuricaemia, 231
Hyperventilation,
  in Reye's syndrome, 120
  in salicylate poisoning, 119
Hypocalcaemia, 125
Hypogammaglobulinaemia, X-linked, 223, 224
Hypoglycaemia,
  asymptomatic, 148
  at night, in diabetes, 133
  in fructosaemia, 201
  in galactosaemia, 200
  in premature infant, *30*, 148
  in Reye's syndrome, 120
  in sepsis, 200
  in Somogyi effect, 133
  neonatal, 231
    causes, 231
  symptomatic, 148
Hypokalaemia,
  in chronic renal failure, 117
  in Fanconi syndrome, 194
  in neuroblastoma, 129
  in salicylate poisoning, 119
  periodic, 117
Hyponatraemia,
  in congenital adrenal hypoplasia, 113
  neonatal, *88–89*, 222
Hypophosphataemia, *12*, 125
Hypopituitarism, *2*, 112
  androgen production defect, 136
Hyporeflexia, 54, 179
Hyposplenism, 128
Hypotension, postural, 17, 131
Hypothalamic tumour, *83–84*, 217–218
Hypothalamus, in tuberculous meningitis, 161
Hypothalamus/pituitary axis,
  assessment, 112–113
  space-occupying lesion, 83–84, 112, 217–218
Hypovolaemia, 131

Ileitis, tuberculous, 189
Imipramine, 137
Immunodeficiency, 233
  hypogammaglobulinaemia, 223, 224
  severe combined (SCID), *90–91*, 223–224
Immunoglobulin A (IgA), deficiency, 47, 172–173, 223
Immunoglobulin E (IgE), in food allergy, 173
Immunoglobulin G (IgG), deficiency, 223
Immunoglobulin M (IgM) deficiency, 223
Immunoglobulin(s), in immune deficiency, 223
Inborn errors of metabolism, 198 (*see also individual disorders*)
Incontinence, urine, 37
  ectopic ureter, *102*, 240–241
Indomethacin, 107, 248
Infection, (*see also individual infections*)
  of frontal sinus, *56–57*, 183
  in acute pericarditis, *98*, 236
  in chronic granulomatous disease, *33*, 153
  in endocardium of right ventricle, *48–49*, 174–175
  in premature infant, 148
  intrauterine, 206
    haemolysis in, 134
  recurrent, in immune deficiency, *90–91*, 223–224

Infection – *continued*
  respiratory tract, (*see* Respiratory tract infections)
  urinary tract, (*see* Urinary tract infection)
Inguinal mass, 42, 165
Inhalation,
  of foreign object, *62–63*, 190–191, 245
  palatal, pharyngeal incoordination, 229
  recurrent, causes, 229
Insulin,
  overdose, 188
  Somogyi effect, *18*, 133
  tolerance test, 112
Intestinal mucosal infarctions, 189
Intracranial lesion, 198
Intracranial pressure,
  raised, 198
    in astrocytoma, medulloblastoma, 204
    in disseminated CNS malignancy, *50–51*, 175–176
    in lead encephalopathy, 121, 123
    in pseudotumour cerebri, 170–171
    VIth nerve palsy, 175
  reduction, 170
Intrauterine growth retardation, 179
Intravenous pyelogram (IVP),
  in ectopic ureter, 241
  in obstructed infected kidney, 124
Intraventricular haemorrhage (IVH), *43*, 149, 166
Intussusception, chronic, 182
Ischaemia of lower limbs, 18, 132

Jaundice,
  cholestatic, *91*, 225
  in galactosaemia, 200
  in G6PD deficiency, *93*, 227
  in typhoid, 219
Jejunal biopsy, 173, 186, 198
Jejunal juice aspiration, 173

Kidney, (*see also* Renal)
  abnormalities, 42, 165
  maturation, 222
  obstructed infected, *9*, 123–124
  scans, 124
Knee, monoarticular arthritis, *1*, 109
Krabbe's leucodystrophy, 179, 180
Kugelberg-Welander disease, 215

Lactic acidosis, 198
Lactose intolerance, 186–187
Lafora body disease, 127
Larva migrans, visceral, 192
Laryngotracheobronchitis, 245
Lassa fever, 219
Lazy leucocyte syndrome, 153
Lead encephalopathy, *8*, 121–123
  differential diagnosis, 122–123
Lead poisoning, 195
  vs. acute intermittent porphyria, 195, 196
  from surma, 150
Legionnaire's disease, 243–244
Lens, dislocation, 237
Lethargy,
  in haemolytic uraemic syndrome, *36*, 158
  in hyperammonaemia, 198
  in pyloric stenosis, *67*, 197
  in pyonephrosis, *9*
Letterer-Siwe disease, 163 (*see also* Histiocytosis X)
Leucopenia, 219
Leukaemia,
  acute lymphoblastic (ALL), *29–30*, 145–147
    CNS involvement, 176
    dermatomyositis associated with, *70*, 202
    markers, 146
Leukodystrophy,
  Krabbe's, 179, 180
  metachromatic, 126
  Perlizaeus-Merzbacher, 179, 180–181
Limb-girdle,
  muscles in dermatomyositis, *70*, 202
  muscular dystrophy, *81–82*, 203, 214–215
Liver biopsy, 92, 225
Löffler's syndrome, 191
Lung,
  collapse, foreign object inhalation, 190
  hyperinflation, 63, 190
Lung disease, chronic suppurative, *75–77*, 209–210
Lymph node biopsy, 146
Lymphoma,
  cervical lymphadenopathy in, 146
  non-Hodgkins, 146, 175–176
    CNS involvement, 176
Lymphopenia, 224

McCune-Albright's syndrome, *35*, 155–157
Malabsorption,
  in rickets, 177
  syndrome, 217
Malrotation, bowel, 142
  intermittent volvulus with, *25–27*, 142
Mantoux test, 160
Marfan's syndrome, *99–100*, 237–238
Measles,
  antibody, 126
  subacute sclerosing panencephalitis, *12–13*, 126–127
Meconium,
  ileus, 185
  peritonitis, 185
Medulloblastoma, *71–73*, 176, 203–205
Melaena, 189
Melanocyte stimulating hormone (MSH), 136
Meningeal spread of systemic disease, 161
Meningitis, 119, 122
  acute hemiplegia in, 145
  in inhalation of foreign object, 190
  pneumococcal, *13–14*, 127–128
  tuberculous (TBM), *37–38*, 123, 159–161
  with urinary tract infection, *10*, 124
Mental retardation,
  in diabetes insipidus, 233
  lead poisoning, 121, 122
Methocholine, 180
Methylmalonic acidaemia, 198
Methylumbelliferylguanidinebenzoate (MUGB) reactive proteases, 185
Micturating cystourethrogram (MCU), 241
Micturition, ectopic ureter, *102*, 240–241
Migraine, *74–75*, 187, 208–209
  classic, 208
  hemiplegic, 145, 208
Mitral regurgitation, 247
Motor seizures, minor, 126
Munchausen's syndrome by proxy, 138, 161
Muscle,
  biopsy, 202, 215
  weakness,
    in dermatomyositis, *70*, 202
    in limb-girdle muscular dystrophy, *81*, 214
Muscular dystrophy,
  limb-girdle, *81–82*, 203, 214–215
  pseudohypertrophic (Duchenne), 203, 214
  vs. dermatomyositis, 203
Mycoplasma pneumoniae infection, *103–104*, 242–244
  complications, 244
Myeloperoxidase deficiency, 154
Myopathies,
  acquired, 214
  acute myoglobinuric, 215
  benign congenital, 214
  of metabolic bone disease, 215
Myositis, *70–71*, 202, 203

NADPH, in fluorescent spot test, 228
Naphthalene, 227
Necrosis, aseptic, 109
Nephritis, shunt, 175
Nephrostomy, 124
Nephrotic syndrome, 17–18, 131–132
Nephroureterectomy, 241
Neuroblastoma, *15–16*, 129–130, 176
  in utero, 130
  staging, 130
Neurofibromatosis, 155, 156
Neurological symptoms,
  drug-induced, *22*, 137–138
  in acute intermittent porphyria, *66*, 196
  in carbamazepine toxicity, *59*, 188
  in disseminated CNS malignancy, *51*, 175–176
  in Riley-Day syndrome, *53*, 179
Neutrophil,
  chemotaxis defects, 153
  defective, 152–153
  function tests, 154
  ingestion disorders, 154
  opsonization defects, 153
Nitroblue tetrazolium (NBT) test, 153
Nystagmus, congenital, 83–84, 217

Oedema,
  angioneurotic, 245
  cerebral, *57*, 171, 183
  in dermatomyositis, *70*, 202
Oesophageal peristalsis, abnormal, 230
Oesophageal stricture, *94–95*, 229
Opsonization defects, 153
Optic atrophy, 217

Organic aciduria, 198
Osteoma, osteoid, 116
Osteomyelitis, 223
  in chronic granulomatous disease, 152
  Salmonella, *13–14*, 127, 128
  vs. sickle-cell disease, 110
Osteoporosis,
  in juvenile chronic arthritis, 116
  in tuberculous arthritis, 115
Otitis media, 45
  pseudotumour cerebri, *45–46*, 170–172
Ovarian cysts, 156
  tumours, 182
Owl eye cells, 207
Oxytocin, 222

Pain,
  abdominal,
    in acute intermittent porphyria, *66*, 195, 208
    in migraine, *74–75*, 208
    in nephrotic syndrome, 17, 131
    in psychogenic polydipsia, *5*, 118
    in typhoid, *85*, 219
    in Wilson's disease, chronic active hepatitis, *77–78*, 212
    sickle-cell crisis, 128
  bone,
    in leukaemia, 146
    in neuroblastoma, 130
  chest, in aortic stenosis, 247
  in limb-girdle muscular dystrophy, *81*, 214
  in muscles, 215
  in poliomyelitis, *87*, 221
  neck, in acute pericarditis, *98–99*, 235
Palatal incoordination, 229
Palsy, cranial nerve, (*see* Cranial nerve palsy)
Panencephalitis, subacute sclerosing (SSPE), *12–13*, 126–127
Papilloedema,
  in disseminated CNS malignancy, 176
  in pseudotumour cerebri, *45*, 170–171
Paraplegia, in chronic granulomatous disease, 34, 154
Paralysis,
  acute, 27–28, 143–145
  in Guillain-Barré syndrome, 220
  in poliomyelitis, 220
Parathormone, 125

Paratyphoid fever, 219
Paresis, in varicella encephalitis, *31*, 150–151
Paroxysmal cold haemoglobinuria, 228
Paroxysmal nocturnal haemoglobinuria (PNH), 228
Pectus excavatum, 100, 237
Pelvic appendix abscess, *55–56*, 182
Pelviureteric junction, obstruction, 124
Penicillin, in pneumococcal meningitis, *14*, 127, 128
Pericardial rub, *99*, 235
Pericardial tap, 236
Pericardiotomy, 236
Pericarditis, acute, *98–99*, 235–236
  idiopathic, 236
Peripheral neuropathy, 221
Peritonitis,
  in nephrotic syndrome, 131
  meconium, 185
Perlizaeus-Merzbacher leukodystrophy, 179, 180–181
Perthes' disease, *4*, 115
  differential diagnosis, 115–116
Pertussis, 75, 185, 210
Pharyngeal incoordination, 229
Pharyngeal pouch, 229
Phenobarbitone,
  in vitamin-D deficient rickets, *11*, 125
Pica, 121
Pitressin, 118
Pituitary hormone, deficiencies, *2*, 112
Platelets,
  antibodies to, 239, 240
  transfusions, 239
Pneumococcal antigen vaccination, 169
Pneumococcal infections, after splenectomy, 169
Pneumococcal meningitis, *13–14*, 127–128
Pneumocystis carinii, 224
Pneumonia,
  atypical, 242
  congenital, 148
  Mycoplasma pneumoniae, *103–104*, 242–244
  severe lobar, 244
Pneumothorax, 166
Poliomyelitis, *87–88*, 220–221
  paralytic, 150
Polydipsia,
  in diabetes insipidus, 233

primary, 234
psychogenic, *5*, 117–118, 234
Polymyositis, 214
  vs. dermatomyositis, 203
  vs. limb-girdle muscular dystrophy, 214
Polyuria,
  causes, 234
  in chronic renal failure, 117
  in Fanconi syndrome, 195
  in nephrogenic diabetes insipidus, 233
  in psychogenic polydipsia, *5*, 117
Porphobilinogen, 196
Porphyria,
  acute intermittent, *66–67*, 195–196
  peripheral neuropathy in, 221
  variegata, 195, 196
  vs. migraine, 208
Postencephalitis syndromes, 179
Postictal state, 139, 140
Post-pericardiotomy syndrome, 236
Potassium, (*see also* Hypokalaemia)
  in congenital adrenal hypoplasia, 113
  loss, in Fanconi syndrome, 194
  theophylline, digoxin effect, 216
Prematurity,
  apnoea of, *30*, 149
  haemoglobin drop in, 19, 134
  hypoglycaemia in, *30*, 148
  hyponatraemia in, *89*, 222
  intraventricular haemorrhage in, *43*, 166
  vitamin E deficiency in, *19*, 134
Propionic acidaemia, 198
Proptosis, 40, 163
Protease inhibitor (Pi) system in α_1-antitrypsin deficiency, 212, 226
Protein enteropathy, cows' milk, (*see* Cows' milk)
Proteinuria, 17, 131
Prothrombin time, 158
Protoporphyrin, free erythrocyte (FEP), 122
Pseudohypoaldosteronism, 114
Pseudotumour cerebri, *45–46*, 170–172
  diseases associated with, 171, 200
Pseudovitamin D deficiency, *51–53*, 177–178
Psittacosis, 243
Psychosis, acute, 126
Psychosocial deprivation, *84*, 217

Puberty, 112
  constitutional delay in, 112
  delayed, 2, 112
  precocious, *35*, 155–157
    central, 156
    peripheral, 156–157
Pulmonary atresia, *107–108*, 248–249
Pulmonary haemorrhage, 166
Pulmonary hypertension, *80*, 213
Pulse,
  in aortic stenosis, *106*, 247
  paradoxical, *98*, 235
Purpura, idiopathic thrombocytopenic (ITP), 239
Pyloric stenosis, *67–68*, 197
Pyonephrosis, *9*, 123–124
Pyrexia,
  in acute pericarditis, *98*, 235
  in erythema multiforme, *24*, 141
  in lead poisoning, 122
  in nephrogenic diabetes insipidus, *97*, 232–233
  in pneumococcal meningitis, *14–15*
  in space-occupying lesions, 122
  of unknown origin (PUO), 219
Pyuria, in ectopic ureter, 241

Q fever, 243

Rash,
  in congenital CMV infection, 207
  in congenital toxoplasmosis, 206
  in dermatomyositis, *70*, 202
  in erythema multiforme, *24*, 141
  in Hand-Schüller-Christian disease, *40*, 163
  in Letterer-Siewe disease, 163
Rectal bleeding, 61, 189
Rehydration,
  in hypovolaemia, 131
  in intermittent volvulus, malrotation, *26–27*, 142
Renal failure, chronic, 117
Renal impairment,
  in haemolytic uraemic syndrome, 158
  rickets with, 125
Renal involvement,
  in bacterial endocarditis, 175
  in Fanconi syndrome, *64–65*, 193–194
Renal tubular acidosis, 178, 194

Renal tubular defects,
  cystinosis, 194–195
  in nephrogenic diabetes insipidus, 233-234
  in rickets, 178
Respiratory distress syndrome, 148
  vs. group B haemolytic streptococcus, 149
Respiratory tract infections,
  acute, *104–105*, 245
  acute pericarditis, *98*, 235–236
  chronic suppurative lung disease, *75–76*, 209–210
  cyanotic episodes, enlarged adenoids, *79–80*, 213
  in haemolytic uraemic syndrome, *36*
  in Reye's syndrome, *7*, 120
  recurrent, 229
    in SCID, *90–91*, 223
  with Perthe's disease, *4*, 115
Reticulocytosis, 227
Retinal detachment, 100, 237
Retinoblastoma, 63
Reye's syndrome, *7*, 119–120
Rhabdomyosarcoma, 176
Rheumatic fever, 110, 236
Rheumatoid arthritis, 110
Rickets,
  hypophosphataemic, 178
  in Fanconi syndrome, *65*, 193, 194
  vitamin-D deficient, *11*, 125
  vitamin-D resistant, *51–53*, 177–178
Riley-Day syndrome, *53–54*, 179–180
Rose Bengal dye, 226
Rubella, congenital, 206

Salicylate poisoning, 119
Salmonella osteomyelitis, *13–14*, 127, 128
Salmonella typhi, 219
Salt-losing crisis, 20, 135, 136
Schumm test, 228
Severe combined immune deficiency (SCID), *90–91*, 223–224
Shigella dysentery, 219
Shunt nephritis, 175
'Sick-cell' syndrome, 113
Sickle-cell disease,
  cerebral haemorrhage in, 144
  crisis, 128, 189
  homozygous, *1–2*, 61, 109, 189
  pneumococcal meningitis with, *13–14*, 127–128
  rectal bleeding with, 61, 189
  Salmonella osteomyelitis with, 128
Sinusitis, frontal, *56–57*, 183
Skeletal survey,
  in acute lymphoblastic leukaemia, 146
  in Hand-Schüller-Christian disease, 163
  in McCune-Albright's syndrome, 155, 156
  multiple fractures in non-accidental injury, *39*, 162
Skin, in porphyria, 196 (*see also* Rash)
Sodium, (*see also* Hypernatraemia; Hyponatraemia)
  in 'sick-cell' syndrome, 113
  in sweat test, 185, 210
Sodium chloride infusion, 118
Somogyi effect, *18*, 132–133
Space-occupying lesion, 122 (*see also* Abscess; *individual tumours*)
  acute hemiplegia with, 145
  cerebellar, *71–73*, 204–205
  hypothalamic/pituitary, 112
  vs. lead encephalopathy, 122
  vs. tuberculous meningitis, 160
Spherocytes, 227
Spina bifida, 11–12, 125
Spinal cord lesion, *33–34*, 154
Spinal muscular atrophy, 215
Splenectomy, 169
Staphylococcal infection, 110
Stature,
  small, 2, 40, 112
  tall,
    in Marfan's syndrome, homocystinuria, *100*, 237
    precocious puberty, *35*, 156
Steinberg's sign, 237, 238
Steroids,
  in thrombocytopenia, 239
  urinary, 113, 114, 136
Steven-Johnson syndrome, 141
Still's disease, 116, 147
Stool,
  in Crohn's disease, 189
  microscopy, 173
Streptococcal infection,
  group B haemolytic, 148–149
  rheumatic fever, 110
  transient synovitis of hip, 115
Subacute sclerosing panencephalitis (SSPE), *12–13*, 126–127

Subdural empyema, 183–184
Subdural haemorrhage, 139, 145, 170
Suicide attempts, *59–60*, 187–188
Sulphonamides, 227
Sweat test, 185, 210
Synovitis, transient of hip, 115
Systemic lupus erythematosus, 215

Tachycardia, supraventricular, 22, 138
Tear, diminished production, 53, 179, 180
Telangiectasia, on nailbed, 202
Temper tantrums, 53, 179
Testes,
   in delayed puberty, 112
   responsiveness to hCG, 113
   strangulated, torted, 165
   undescended, 165
β-Thalassaemia major, *44–45*, 167–169
Theophylline, 82, 216
Thrombocytopenia,
   causes, in neonate, 239
   idiopathic thrombocytopenic
      purpura, 239
   in haemolytic uraemic syndrome, 158
   isoimmune, *100–101*, 239–240
Thrombosis,
   acute hemiplegia, *27–28*, 144
   arterial, in nephrotic syndrome, 132
   in homocystinuria, 238
   non-septic, of lateral venous sinus, 170
   renal vein, 132
   superficial venous cerebral, 183
Thrombus, fibrin, 158
Tonsils, enlarged, *79–80*, 213
TORCH antibodies, 230
Toxicological screen, 137, 140
Toxocara antibody test, 192
Toxocara canis infestations, *63–64*, 192
Toxocara skin test, 192
Toxoplasma gondii, congenital infection, 206
Tracheo-oesophageal cleft, 229
Tracheo-oesophageal fistula, *94–95*, 229–230
Transposition of great vessels, 248
Trephine biopsy, 146
Trichinosis, 203, 215
Tricuspid atresia, 248
Tuberculosis,
   abscess on chest wall, 152
   acute pericarditis in, 236
Tuberculous arthritis, 115

Tuberculous ileitis, 189
Tuberculous meningitis (TBM), *37–38*, 123, 159–161
Typhoid, *85–86*, 219

Ulcerative colitis, 111, 189
Uraemia, in congenital adrenal
   hypoplasia, 113
Ureter, abnormal, 42, 165
   ectopic, low-placed, *101–102*, 240–241
Ureteral obstruction, *9*, 123–124
Ureteric buds, 241
Urethral stricture, 78
Urethrogram, micturating (MCU), 241
Urinary tract infection,
   inguinal mass with, 165
   in pyonephrosis, 124
Urine,
   11 oxygenation index, 136
   retention, 77, 78
     in pelvic appendix abscess, *55*, 182
   steroids in, 113, 114, 136
   test, for Somogyi effect, 133
Urticaria, 141

Vaginal bleeding, 35, 155
Vanillylmandelic acid (VMA), 180
Varicella encephalitis, *31–32*, 150–151
Vasoactive intestinal peptide (VIP), 129
Vasoconstriction, pulmonary, 213
Ventilation, 43
   positive pressure, 43, 166
Ventricle, right, endocardium infection, *48–49*, 174
Ventricle, third, astrocytoma, 204, 218
Ventricular hypertrophy, right, 80, 213
Ventricular septum, in pulmonary
   atresia, *107–108*, 248–249
Vertebral bodies, collapse, *34*, 154
Virilization, female, 137
Viruses, infections,
   encephalitis, 122, 160, 171
   in acute encephalopathy, 221
   in acute pericarditis, 236
   in aplastic anaemia, 146, 147
   in erythema multiforme, 141
   in Reye's syndrome, 120
   respiratory, laryngotracheo-
      bronchitis, 245
   vs. dermatomyositis, 203
Vitamin D,
   deficient rickets, 125

Vitamin D, – *continued*
resistant rickets, *51–53*, 177–178
supplements, 125, 194
Vitamin E deficiency, *19*, 134–135
Volvulus,
intermittent, with malrotation, *25–27*, 142
without malrotation, 142
Vomiting,
hyponatraemia, hyperkalaemia in, 113
in astrocytoma, medulloblastoma, *71–72*, 204
in congenital adrenal hypoplasia, *3*
in diabetes insipidus, *96–97*, 233
in galactosaemia, fructosaemia, *69*, 199–201
in hypovolaemia, nephrotic syndrome, 17, 131
in labour, neonatal hyponatraemia, *89*, 222
in malrotation with intermittent volvulus, *25–27*, 142
in migraine, *75*, 208
in pseudotumour cerebri, *45*
in pyloric stenosis, *67–68*, 197
in pyonephrosis, *9*, 124
paroxysmal cough with, 185
Von Gierke's disease, *95–96*, 231

Water,
deprivation test, 117–118, 234
fresh, drowning, 139
Weil-Felix reaction, 243
Wheezing,
acute epiglottitis, *104*, 245
foreign object inhalation, *62*, 190
White blood cell (WBC),
count,
in Reye's syndrome, 120
in vitamin E deficiency, haemolysis, *19*, 134
transfusions, 154
Widal's agglutination test, 219
Wilson's disease, 126, 212
Wiskott-Aldrich syndrome, 223

Xanthines, actions, 216
X-ray,
chest,
in acute pericarditis, 236
in chronic suppurative lung disease, 209
in inhalation of foreign object, *63*
in *Mycoplasma pneumoniae* infection, 243
in tuberculous meningitis, 160
in typhoid, 219
lateral neck, 245
skull,
hypothalamic tumours, 218
intracerebral calcification, 206
Xylose absorption, 187

Yersinia enterocolitica infections, 182, 219

Ziehl-Nielsen stain, 160